BLUEPR
UROLO

CW00329544

BLUEPRINTS
UROLOGY

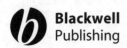

Blackwell Publishing, Inc., 350 Main Street, Malden, Massachusetts
02148-5018, USA
Blackwell Publishing Ltd, 9600 Garsington Road, Oxford OX4 2DQ, UK
Blackwell Publishing Asia Pty Ltd, 550 Swanston Street, Carlton, Victoria
3053, Australia

04 05 06 07 5 4 3 2 1

ISBN: 1-4051-0400-7

Library of Congress Cataloging-in-Publication Data

Zaslau, Stanley.
  Blueprints urology / Stanley Zaslau.
      p. ; cm. — (Blueprints)
  Includes index.
  ISBN 1-4051-0400-7 (pbk.)
  1. Urology—Handbooks, manuals, etc.
  [DNLM: 1. Urogenital Diseases—Handbooks. 2. Urogenital Diseases—
Outlines. 3. Urologic Diseases—Handbooks. 4. Urologic Diseases—
Outlines. WJ 18.2 Z35b 2004] I. Title. II. Series.

RC872.9.Z37 2004
616.6–dc22

                                                         2004003925

A catalogue record for this title is available from the British Library

Acquisitions: Beverly Copland
Development: Selene Steneck
Production: Debra Murphy
Cover design: Hannus Design Associates
Interior design: Mary McKeon
Illustrations: Electronic Illustrators Group
Typesetter: International Typesetting and Composition, Fort Lauderdale, FL
Printed and bound by Capital City Press, Ann Arbor, MI

For further information on Blackwell Publishing, visit our website:
www.blackwellmedstudent.com

Notice: The indications and dosages of all drugs in this book have been recommended in the medical literature and conform to the practices of the general community. The medications described do not necessarily have specific
approval by the Food and Drug Administration for use in the diseases and
dosages for which they are recommended. The package insert for each drug
should be consulted for use and dosage as approved by the FDA. Because
standards for usage change, it is advisable to keep abreast of revised recommendations, particularly those concerning new drugs.

Contents

Chapter 8: Genitourinary Oncology

Contributors

Associate Editor
Jay Singh, DO
Resident
Brookdale University Medical Center
Brooklyn, New York

Student Editors
Jill Yeager
Class of 2004
West Virginia University
Morgantown, West Virginia

Brian DeFade
Class of 2004
West Virginia School of Osteopathic Medicine
Lewisburg, West Virginia

Reviewers

Sean Armin, MD
1st year resident - Neurosurgery
Loma Linda University
Los Angeles, California

James Fletcher, MD
Class of 2003
Eastern Virginia Medical School
Norfolk, Virginia

Henry Hwang, MD
Intern, Department of Surgery
University of Michigan Medical School
Ann Arbor, Michigan

Chad A. Peterson, MD
1st year resident, Urologic Surgery
Oregon Health and Science University
Portland, Oregon

Sarah Kathleen Taylor
Class of 2004
Baylor College of Medicine
Houston, Texas

Preface

Blueprints have become the standard for medical students to use during their clerkship rotations and sub-internships and as a review book before taking the USMLE Steps 2 and 3.

Blueprints initially were only available for the five main specialties: medicine, pediatrics, obstetrics and gynecology, surgery, and psychiatry. Students found these books so valuable that they asked for Blueprints in other topics and so family medicine, emergency medicine, neurology, cardiology, and radiology were added.

In an effort to answer a need for high yield review books for the elective rotations, Blackwell Publishing now brings you Blueprints in pocket size. These books are developed to provide students in the shorter, elective rotations—often taken in 4th year—with the same high yield, essential contents of the larger Blueprints books. These new pocket-sized Blueprints will be invaluable for those students who need to know the essentials of a clinical area but were unable to take the rotation. Students in physician assistant, nurse practitioner, and osteopath programs will find these books meet their needs for the clinical specialties.

Feedback from student reviewers gives high praise for this addition to the Blueprints brand. Each of these new books was developed to be read in a short time period and to address the basics needed during a particular clinical rotation. Please see the Series Page for a list of the books that will soon be in your bookstore.

Acknowledgments

I would like to thank my contributing authors for their enthusiasm and their effort. I appreciate the many helpful suggestions and critique given by our reviewers. A very heartfelt thanks to Beverly Copland for allowing this idea to develop from a brief course syllabus to an impressive subject review. Thanks to a great editor, Selene Steneck, whose support and assistance has been much appreciated from inception to completion of the book. Thanks to my students and residents, whose interest and enthusiasm for urology fuels my passion to continue on as an educator. Finally, a special thank you to the most important people: my wife, April, and my son, Darren, whose everlasting love and support make my goals attainable.

—Stanley Zaslau

Abbreviations

AFP	α-Fetoprotein
AML	Angiomyolipoma
ART	Assisted reproductive technique
ASA	Antisperm antibodies
AUA	American Urologic Association
BCG	Bacille Calmette-Guérin
BOO	Bladder outlet obstruction
BPH	Benign prostatic hyperplasia
BTA	Bladder tumor antigen
BUN	Blood urea nitrogen
CBAVD	Congenital bilateral absence of the vas deferens
CBC	Complete blood count
CIS	Carcinoma in situ
CP-CPPS	Chronic prostatitis/chronic pelvic pain syndrome
CT	Computed tomography
CVA	Costovertebral angle
DHT	Dihydrotestosterone
DI	Detrusor instability
DMSO	Dimethylsulfoxide
DRE	Digital rectal examination
DSD-DH	Detrusor sphincter dyssynergia with detrusor hyperreflexia
ED	Erectile dysfunction
EPN	Emphysematous pyelonephritis
EPS	Expressed prostatic secretions
ESR	Erythrocyte sedimentation rate
ESRD	End-stage renal disease
ESWL	Extracorporeal shock-wave lithotripsy
5AR	5-alpha reductase
FNA	Fine-needle aspiration
FSD	Female sexual dysfunction
FSFI	Female Sexual Function Index
FSH	Follicle-stimulating hormone
FTA-ABS	Fluorescent treponemal antibody absorption (test)
GC	Gonococcal urethritis
GI	Granuloma inguinale
GIFT	Gamete intrafallopian transfer
GMP	Guanosine monophosphate
GnRH	Gonadotrophin-releasing hormone

hCG	Human chorionic gonadotrophin
HIFU	High-intensity focused ultrasound
HPRCC	Hereditary papillary renal cell carcinoma
HPV	Human papilloma virus
HRT	Hormone replacement therapy
IC	Interstitial cystitis
ICSI	Intracytoplasmic sperm injection
IIEF	International Index of Erectile Function
IVC	Inferior vena cava
IVF	In vitro fertilization
IVP	Intravenous pyelogram
KUB	Kidneys, ureters, bladder
LDH	Lactate dehydrogenase
LFT	Liver function test
LH	Luteinizing hormone
LMN	Lower motor neuron
LUTS	Lower urinary tract symptoms
MAOI	Monoamine oxidase inhibitor
MAP	Magnesium ammonium phosphate
MCC	Micturition control center
MESA	Microepididymal sperm aspiration
MPG	Mercaptopropionyl glycine
NGU	Nongonococcal urethritis
NMP	Nuclear matrix protein
NO	Nitric oxide
NOS	Nitric oxide synthase
NPT	Nocturnal penile tumescence
NSAID	Nonsteroidal anti-inflammatory drug
NSGCT	Nonseminomatous germ cell tumor
PCNL	Percutaneous nephrolithotomy
PD	Peyronie's disease
PESA	Percutaneous epididymal sperm aspiration
PID	Pelvic inflammatory disease
PIN	Prostate intraepithelial neoplasia
PMC	Pontine micturition center
PNM	Polymorphonuclear leukocyte
PSA	Prostate-specific antigen
PTH	Parathyroid hormone
PVR	Postvoiding residual
RBC	Red blood cell
RCC	Renal cell carcinoma
RF	Radiofrequency
RH	Renal hypercalciuria
RPF	Retroperitoneal fibrosis
RPG	Retrograde pyelogram
RPLND	Retroperitoneal lymph node dissection
RPR	Rapid plasma reagin (test)
RUG	Retrograde urethrography

SCC	Squamous cell carcinoma
SHBG	Sex hormone binding globulin
SLE	Systemic lupus erythematosus
SSRI	Selective serotonin reuptake inhibitor
STD	Sexually transmitted disease
TCC	Transitional cell carcinoma
TMP-SMX	Trimethoprim-sulfamethoxazole
TPN	Total parental nutrition
TRUS	Transrectal ultrasound
TS	Tuberous sclerosis
TUIP	Transurethral incision of the prostate
TUMT	Transurethral microwave thermotherapy
TUNA	Transurethral needle ablation
TURBT	Transurethral resection of bladder tumor
TURP	Transurethral resection of the prostate
UDS	Urodynamic studies
UMN	Upper motor neuron
UPJ	Ureteropelvic junction
US	Ultrasound
UTI	Urinary tract infection
UVJ	Ureterovesical junction
VCUG	Voiding cystourethrogram
VDRL	Venereal Disease Research Laboratory (test)
VHL	Von Hippel-Lindau syndrome
VUR	Vesicoureteral reflux
XGP	Xanthogranulomatous pyelonephritis
XRT	External beam radiotherapy

Normal Lab Values

Blood, Plasma, Serum

Alanine aminotransferase (ALT, GPT at 30°C)	8–20 U/L
Alpha-fetoprotein (AFP)	0–10 ng/mL
Amylase, serum	25–125 U/L
Aspartate aminotransferase (AST, GOT at 30°C)	8–20 U/L
Bilirubin, serum (adult)	
Total	0.1–1.0 mg/dL
Direct	0.0–0.3 mg/dL
Calcium, serum (Ca^{2+})	8.4–10.2 mg/dL
Cholesterol, serum	Recommended: <200 mg/dL
Cortisol, serum	
0800 h	5–23 ng/dL
1600 h	3–15 ng/dL
2000 h	≤50% of 0800 h
Creatine kinase, serum	
Male	25–90 U/L
Female	10–70 U/L
Creatinine, serum	0.6–1.2 mg/dL
Electrolytes, serum	
Sodium (Na^+)	136–145 mEq/L
Chloride (Cl^-)	95–105 mEq/L
Potassium (K^+)	3.5–5.0 mEq/L
Bicarbonate (HCO_3^-)	22–28 mEq/L
Magnesium (Mg^{2+})	1.5–2.0 mEq/L
Ferritin, serum	
Male	15–200 ng/mL
Female	12–150 ng/mL
Follicle-stimulating hormone, serum/plasma	
Male	4–25 mIU/mL
Female	
Premenopause	4–30 mIU/mL
Midcycle peak	10–90 mIU/mL
Postmenopause	40–250 mIU/mL

Gases, arterial blood (room air)

    pH   7.35–7.45

    P_{CO_2} 33–45 mm Hg

    P_{O_2} 75–105 mm Hg

Glucose, serum

    Fasting   70–110 mg/dL

    2-h postprandial   <120 mg/dL

Growth hormone-arginine stimulation

    Fasting   <5 ng/mL

    Provocative stimuli   >7 ng/mL

Human chorionic gonadotropin (hCG)   <5 mIU/mL

Iron   50–70 µg/dL

Lactate dehydrogenase, serum   45–90 U/L

Luteinizing hormone, serum/plasma

    Male   6–23 mIU/mL

    Female

        Follicular phase   5–30 mIU/mL

        Midcycle   75–150 mIU/mL

        Postmenopause   30–200 mIU/mL

Osmolality, serum   275–295 mOsm/kg H_2O

Parathyroid hormone, serum, N-terminal   230–630 pg/mL

Phosphate (alkaline), serum (*p*-NPP at 30°C)   20–70 µ/L

Phosphorus (inorganic), serum   3.0–4.5 mg/dL

Prolactin, serum (hPRL)   <20 ng/mL

Proteins, serum

    Total (recumbent)   6.0–7.8 g/dL

    Albumin   3.5–5.5 g/dL

    Globulin   2.3–3.5 g/dL

Prostate-specific antigen   0–4 ng/mL

Testosterone, serum   300–1000 ng/dL

Thyroid-stimulating hormone, serum

    or plasma   0.5–5.0 nU/mL

Thyroidal iodine (^{123}I) uptake   8%–30% of administered dose per 24 h

Thyroxine (T_4), serum   5–12 ng/dL

Triglycerides, serum   35–160 mg/dL

Triiodothyronine (T_3), serum (RIA)   115–190 ng/dL

Triiodothyronine (T_9), resin uptake   25%–35%

Urea nitrogen, serum (BUN)   7–18 mg/dL

Uric acid, serum   3.0–8.2 mg/dL

Hematologic

Bleeding time (template)   2–7 min

Erythrocyte count

    Male   4.3–5.9 million/mm^3

    Female   3.5–5.5 million/mm^3

Erythrocyte sedimentation rate
(Westergren)
    Male — 0–15 mm/h
    Female — 0–20 mm/h
Hematocrit
    Male — 41%–53%
    Female — 36%–46%
Hemoglobin A_{1C} — ≤6%
Hemoglobin, blood
    Male — 13.5–17.5 g/dL
    Female — 12.0–16.0 g/dL
Leukocyte count and differential
    Leukocyte count — 4500–11,000/mm^3
    Segmented neutrophils — 54%–62%
    Bands — 3%–5%
    Eosinophils — 1%–3%
    Basophils — 0%–0.75%
    Lymphocytes — 25%–33%
    Monocytes — 3%–7%
Mean corpuscular hemoglobin — 25.4–34.6 pg/cell
Mean corpuscular hemoglobin
concentration — 31%–36% Hb/cell
Mean corpuscular volume — 80–100 mm^3
Partial thromboplastin time (activated) — 25–40 s
Platelet count — 150,000–400,000/mm^3
Prothrombin time — 11–15 s
Reticulocyte count — 0.5%–1.5% of red cells
Thrombin time — <2 s deviation from control

Volume
  Plasma
    Male — 25–43 mL/kg
    Female — 28–45 mL/kg
  Red cell
    Male — 20–36 mL/kg
    Female — 19–31 mL/kg

Urine
Calcium — 100–300 mg/24 h
Chloride — Varies with intake
Creatine clearance
    Male — 97–137 mL/min
    Female — 88–128 mL/min
Osmolality — 50–1400 mOsm/kg H_2O
Oxalate — 8–40 ng/mL
Potassium — Varies with diet

Proteins, total	<150 mg/24 h
Sodium	40–220 mEq/24 h
Uric acid	210–750 mg/24 h

Urinalysis

Color	Clear
Odor	None
Glucose	None
Ketones	None
Protein	<150 mg/24 h
pH	4.5–8.0
Specific gravity	1.001–1.035
Red cells	0–3/HPF
White cells	0–3/HPF
Bacteria	Negative
Crystals	Negative
Epithelial cells	Not significant

Seminal Fluid Analysis

Appearance	Opaque, gray-white, highly viscid
Volume	2–5 mL
Liquefaction	Complete within 30 min
pH	7.2–8.0
Leukocytes	Occasional or absent
Count	20–250 million/mL
Motility	50%–80% with progressive active motility
Morphology	50%–90% with normal forms

1

Anatomy and Physiology of the Genitourinary System

ADRENAL GLANDS

The adrenal glands are paired organs located above the kidneys bilaterally. The right adrenal gland is triangular in shape, whereas the left has a more elongated, leaflike appearance. Each adrenal gland is contained within its respective specialized retroperitoneal connective tissue, **Gerota's fascia,** which also contains the kidneys. The adrenal glands are composed of two distinct regions: an outer adrenal cortex, and the inner adrenal medulla. The cortex is composed of three specific layers: the outer zona glomerulosa, the middle zona fasciculata, and the inner zona reticularis. The medulla is composed of chromaffin cells that are derived from the neural crest cells. This region secretes hormones such as epinephrine. The cortex secretes several different hormones, including corticosteroids, androgens, and aldosterone.

Three arteries supply the adrenal gland: the inferior phrenic artery, the aorta, and the renal arteries, which supply the superior, medial, and inferior parts of the gland, respectively. A short vein drains the right adrenal gland into the inferior vena cava directly, whereas the left adrenal vein empties into the left renal vein.

The innervation to the adrenal gland is to the adrenal medulla. Splanchnic nerves and the celiac ganglia send sympathetic fibers, which synapse with the chromaffin cells.

The lymphatics follow the venous drainage and drain into the lateral aortic lymph nodes.

KIDNEYS

The kidneys are paired, bean-shaped organs located in the retroperitoneum and lie in an oblique orientation lateral to the psoas muscle. The right kidney is slightly lower than the left because of the presence of the liver. Each kidney has an approximate weight of 150 g. The right kidney is in close proximity to the duodenum, the liver, and the hepatic flexure. The left kidney is close to the stomach, the pancreas, and the splenic flexure.

The kidneys and the adrenal glands are contained in Gerota's fascia, which protects against the spread of renal infections, fluid extravasation, malignancy, and bleeding from reaching adjacent

1

peritoneal structures. The fatty tissue external to Gerota's fascia is known as the **paranephric fat,** whereas the fat contained within Gerota's fascia is referred to as **perinephric fat.**

The renal artery is typically a single end artery, although there may be two or more arising from the aorta. These extra arteries are referred to as supernumerary arteries. The renal arteries are located posterior to the renal vein and are anterior to the renal pelvis. The renal veins accompany the arteries and empty into the inferior vena cava. The left renal vein is unique in that it receives drainage from the left adrenal veins superiorly, left gonadal veins inferiorly, and lumbar veins posteriorly. The right renal vein, on the other hand, drains directly into the inferior vena cava.

Renal nerves arise from the renal plexus, which overlies the aorta and the preganglionic fibers from the T8 to L2 spinal segments. The nerves accompany the arteries and enter the kidney at the hilum. Parasympathetic innervation is from the vagus nerve. Pain due to distention and stretching of the renal capsule, renal pelvis, or upper ureter is transmitted via the sympathetic fibers.

The renal lymphatics are abundant and follow the renal blood vessels, draining into the para-aortic lymph nodes on the left and into the interaortocaval and right paracaval nodes on the right. The lymphatic drainage from the left para-aortic region can cross and drain into the right-side lymphatic system. This is important in the spread of malignant processes that occur in the retroperitoneum.

Malformations of the kidney are not uncommon. **Renal agenesis** (absence of the kidney) and **renal hypoplasia** (decreased renal size due to fewer than normal number of calices) are examples of renal malformations. In the situation of renal agenesis, the ipsilateral adrenal gland is found in its usual position. One of the more common malformations is fusion of the two kidneys. They may be joined together at their lower ends, referred to as a **horseshoe kidney,** or they may be completely united, forming a **disk kidney.** Kidneys are referred to as **ectopic** when they are found in other regions, such as in the true pelvis.

RENAL PELVIS, CALYCES, AND URETER

The renal collecting system is composed of the renal calices, the renal pelvis, and the ureter. The renal pelvis is made up of 2 or 3 major calyces, which form from 8 to 12 minor calyces from the tips of the renal pyramids. The ureter is approximately 25 to 30 cm long and is a thick-walled, narrow cylindrical tube. It courses downward toward the fundus of the bladder. In females, the ureter travels posterior to the uterine artery; in males, it travels posterior to the vas deferens. The ureter passes through the bladder wall obliquely through the specialized fibromuscular **sheath of Waldeyer**. The ureteral orifice opens into the bladder base in the interureteric ridge of the trigone. Waldeyer's sheath provides a sphincteric mechanism to prevent reflux.

The three areas of relative narrowing of the ureter are the ureteropelvic junction (UPJ), the site of crossing of the iliac vessels, and the ureterovesical junction (UVJ). The narrowest point of the ureter is at the UVJ and measures approximately 1 to 3 mm. These sites of narrowing are important because urinary tract calculi can become lodged in these areas and lead to ureteral obstruction.

The blood supply to the renal pelvis and upper ureter is derived from the renal arteries. The midportion of the ureter obtains its blood supply from the gonadal artery and aorta. The distal portions of the ureter receive blood from branches of the common iliac arteries. The venous drainage of the ureter accompanies the respective arterial supply.

Innervation to the ureter is autonomic and originates from the T10 to L2 levels, whereas the parasympathetic fibers are from the S2 to S4 spinal segment. Visceral pain from distention is referred to the somatic branches relating to the spinal segments.

Congenital anomalies of the ureter include ureteral atresia (absent or blind-ending ureter), duplication of the ureter (complete or incomplete), ureterocele (cystic dilation of the terminal intravesical ureter), ectopic location of the ureteral orifices, and abnormalities of ureteral position. In complete duplication of the ureter, the presence of two ureteral buds leads to the formation of two totally separate ureters and two separate renal pelves.

BLADDER

The bladder is a hollow, muscular organ that serves as a reservoir for the storage and elimination of urine. The average capacity of the adult bladder is approximately 400 to 500 mL. The superior surface is covered by peritoneum, whereas the posterior surface (base) lies on the ventral aspect of the rectum in the male and on the vagina in the female. The potential space between the ventral surface of the bladder and the pubis is the **retropubic of Retzius.** The apex of the bladder is anchored to the umbilicus by a fibrous cord known as the **urachus** (median umbilical ligament). Abnormalities of the urachus can occur, such as patent urachus, which can lead to urine leaking to the umbilicus; and urachal cysts and diverticula, which can become infected. Urachal adenocarcinoma can also result.

The arterial supply of the bladder is extensive and receives contributions from the superior, middle, and inferior vesical arteries. These vessels are derived from the anterior trunk of the hypogastric (internal iliac) artery. In the female, additional branches are derived from the uterine and vaginal arteries. Venous drainage of the bladder is into the hypogastric (internal iliac) veins.

Parasympathetic nerves from S2 to S4 via the pelvic splanchnic nerve supply the detrusor muscle and are active during micturition. The sympathetic innervation is derived from T10 to L2, predominates in the base of the bladder, and is active during urine storage and compliance.

The bladder wall is rich in lymphatics, which drain into the external and common iliac lymph nodes.

PROSTATE

The prostate is a walnut-shaped gland that lies between the neck of the bladder and the external sphincter. It weighs approximately 20 g in the adult. However, in benign prostatic hyperplasia, growth of the glandular component can cause an increase in prostate weight. The prostate is fixed to the pelvic floor by the transversalis fascia and the puboprostatic ligaments. Posteriorly, the prostate is separated from the rectum by Denonvilliers' fascia. Just proximal to the external striated sphincter, the ejaculatory ducts empty posteriorly into the verumontanum into the prostatic urethra. The prostate contains four distinct anatomic zones: peripheral, central, transition, and periurethral. The bulk of the gland is composed of the peripheral zone, which makes up 70% of the volume of the prostate. The central zone accounts for 25% of prostate volume, and the transition zone accounts for 5%.

Primary arterial blood supply to the prostate is derived from the prostatic artery, which is a branch of the inferior vesical artery. Venous drainage is through the periprostatic plexus that drains into the hypogastric veins.

Innervation of the prostate is via the pelvic plexus, with parasympathetic innervation deriving from the pelvic splanchnic nerve and sympathetics from the hypogastric nerve.

Prostatic lymphatics drain primarily into the obturator and internal iliac nodes, with posterior drainage to the presacral lymph nodes.

On digital rectal examination, the prostate's posterior portion can be palpated as well as the seminal vesicles (when they are inflamed or indurated, as seen with advanced prostate cancer). The normal prostate gland has a fleshy feel somewhat similar to that of the muscles of the thenar eminence. Prostatic masses have a nodular or indurated feel. These are considered to be abnormal, and prostate needle biopsy is recommended to determine the presence of prostate cancer.

URETHRA

The male urethra is approximately 21 cm long and is divided into four anatomic divisions: pendulous or penile urethra, bulbar urethra, membranous urethra, and prostatic urethra. The prostatic urethra is also referred to as the posterior urethra and is lined by transitional epithelium, whereas the remainder of the urethra is lined by stratified columnar epithelium and stratified squamous epithelium in the most distal portion.

The blood supply to the urethra is from the bulbourethral artery, a branch of the pudendal artery. The lymphatic drainage of the anterior urethra is into the superficial and deep inguinal nodes. The posterior urethra drains into the pelvic lymph nodes.

The female urethra is approximately 2 to 4 cm long. The distal two-thirds is lined with stratified squamous epithelium, and the proximal one-third is lined with transitional epithelium. The anterior urethra is defined as the distal one-third and drains into the superficial and deep inguinal nodes. The posterior, or proximal two-thirds, drains into the pelvic lymph nodes.

TESTES, EPIDIDYMIDES, VASA DEFERENTIA, AND SEMINAL VESICLES

The testes are paired ovoid structures that reside in the scrotum. Adjacent to the testicle on its posterior aspect is the epididymis. The tunica albuginea, a dense fibrous covering, surrounds the testes. The testis drains into the epididymis, which forms the lumen of the vas deferens (ductus deferens). The vas deferens runs posteriorly in the spermatic cord at the inguinal canal and courses over the ureter and along the base of the bladder. The seminal vesicles are the lateral outpocketings of the vas deferens at the base of the prostate. Spermatozoa are stored in the ampulla of the vas deferens; the seminal vesicles add to the volume of the ejaculate.

Blood supply to the testes and epididymides is from the internal spermatic artery, which arises from the aorta just below the renal arteries. Venous drainage is into the pampiniform plexus and the spermatic vein, which drains into the renal vein on the left and directly into the inferior vena cava on the right.

The lymphatic drainage of the left testis is into the para-aortic lymph nodes that are located primarily between the renal vessels and the bifurcation of the aorta. The lymphatic drainage of the right testis is into the right interaortocaval nodes.

PENIS

The penis is composed of three spongelike tissue bodies: paired corpora cavernosa and the nonerectile corpus spongiosum, which contains the urethra. The penis receives its blood supply from the internal pudendal artery, which divides into a superficial and deep penile artery. The venous drainage is by the deep dorsal vein.

The innervation to the skin and fascia of the penis is via the dorsal nerve, a branch of the pudendal nerve. Erection is mediated by sexual desire and stimulation. This causes nitric oxide release and potentiation of parasympathetic activity that results in relaxation of the cavernosal arterial smooth muscles. This results in increased cavernosal arterial blood flow. The engorgement of the corpora causes compression of venous outflow through emissary veins, leading to rigidity. Ejaculation, on the other hand, occurs due to sympathetic stimulation that leads to contraction of the bladder neck and pelvic muscles and an antegrade flow of the ejaculate volume.

The lymphatic drainage of the penis is to the superficial and deep inguinal lymph nodes, and then to the external iliac lymph nodes.

Urolithiasis and Acquired Obstructive Uropathy

Urolithiasis

■ Epidemiology

Approximately 12% of all individuals will experience kidney stone disease. Males have a threefold increased risk compared with females, although females tend to have a higher proportion of infection-related stones. African Americans have about one-third the incidence of stones in comparison with the Caucasian population. The peak incidence is in the fourth to sixth decades. Renal stones are more common in affluent, industrialized countries and in arid climates.

■ Pathogenesis

Many theories attempt to explain the etiology of kidney stones. In general, two basic factors are necessary for stone formation:

1. Crystal formation and aggregation
2. Deficiency of inhibitor substances

Promoters of stone formation include supersaturation of crystals in the urine, such as calcium, uric acid, cystine, and magnesium ammonium phosphate (struvite); low urine pH; and diet rich in oxalate. In addition, genetic enzymatic disorders such as cystinuria, abnormal purine metabolism as seen in Lesch-Nyhan syndrome, and renal tubular acidosis have been associated with recurrent stone formation.

Urinary inhibitors of stone formation include citrate, magnesium, nephrocalcin, and Tamm-Horsfall protein.

Calcium Stones

Calcium oxalate stones, with or without a calcium phospate component, are the most common type, comprising 70% of all urinary stones, with a recurrence rate of 10% at 1 year and 35% at 5 years. Formation of calcium stones is multifactorial, but the most common underlying cause is hypercalciuria. **Absorptive hypercalciuria (AH)** is the most common form. AH is caused by increased intestinal absorption of calcium and reduced renal tubular reabsorption of calcium due to the suppression of parathyroid hormone (PTH).

Absorptive hypercalciuria is subdivided into three types. AH type I is independent of diet; urinary calcium remains elevated despite a calcium-restricted diet. Conversely, urinary calcium in AH type II is normal with a calcium-controlled diet. AH type III is secondary to a phosphate renal leak. Decreased serum phosphate leads to an increase in 1,25-dihydroxyvitamin D synthesis. This results in increased absorption of phosphate and calcium from the intestine and an increased renal excretion of calcium. Urinary calcium remains elevated on a restricted diet.

Renal hypercalciuria (RH) is caused by impaired renal tubular reabsorption of calcium, which leads to calcium loss and secondary hyperparathyroidism. Normocalcemia, elevated PTH, and high fasting urinary calcium are characteristic of RH.

Resorptive hypercalciuria is caused by primary hyperparathyroidism. Elevated serum and urinary calcium is secondary to elevated PTH secretion, causing excessive bone resorption and an increased absorption of intestinal calcium.

Hyperoxaluric calciuria is most frequently found in patients with inflammatory bowel disease (such as Crohn's disease), small bowel resection, and bowel bypass. Renal calculi develop in 5% to 10% of patients with these conditions. Intestinal fat malabsorption causes calcium to complex with fatty acids in the intestinal lumen. This reduces the normal binding with oxalate and increases oxalate availability for absorption. In addition, poorly absorbed bile salts and fatty acids increase permeability to oxalate in the large bowel. Primary hyperoxaluria is a rare hereditary disorder. It is associated with calcium oxalate renal stones as well as other distant deposits of oxalate. Patients can develop progressive renal failure and eventually die.

Citrate is an inhibitor of urolithiasis. **Hypocitraturic calcium nephrolithiasis** is commonly associated with distal renal tubular acidosis type I, thiazide therapy, and chronic diarrhea. Acidosis enhances citrate reabsorption, whereas alkalosis promotes citrate excretion. RTA type I is characterized by an inability to concentrate urine pH below 5.5, an elevated serum chloride level, and low serum potassium and bicarbonate levels.

Uric Acid Stones

Uric acid stones account for 5% to 10% of all urinary calculi. Uric acid is the end product of purine metabolism and exists in the urine as two forms: uric acid and uric salt. Uric acid is a weak acid and is insoluble if the urine pH is less than 6, whereas uric salt is 20 times more soluble. Three main factors are needed in the formation of uric acid stones: low urine pH, low urinary volume, and hyperuricosuria. Patients with gout, myeloproliferative diseases, and those treated for malignant conditions with cytotoxic drugs have a high incidence of uric acid stones. Patients present with a urinary pH consistently less than 5.5, suggesting the importance of urinalysis in patients with suspected stone disease.

Cystine Stones

Cystine stones make up about 1% of all urinary calculi. Cystine stones are associated with cystinuria, an inherited autosomal recessive defect in renal tubular reabsorption of cystine, ornithine, lysine, and arginine (COLA). The genetic defects associated with cystinuria have been mapped to chromosomes 2p.16 and 19q13.1.

Struvite Stones

A struvite stone is an infectious stone composed of magnesium ammonium phosphate (MAP). Struvite stones constitute about 15% to 20% of all calculi. They are most frequently found in women. *Proteus, Pseudomonas, Klebsiella, Staphylococcus,* and *Mycoplasma* are common infectious etiologies of struvite stones. These organisms split urea and result in an alkaline pH. The typical urinary pH of a patient with a MAP stone is rarely below 7.2. Foreign bodies and neurogenic bladder can also predispose patients to MAP stones.

■ Clinical Manifestations

Signs and Symptoms

Patients with urinary stones often note an acute onset of severe pain. Unlike pain secondary to other abdominal causes, such as peritonitis, patients with urinary calculi are frequently unable to stay still. The type of pain might elucidate the location of the stone. For example, renal stones are associated with pain that localizes to the flank with costovertebral tenderness. Stones in the ureter often cause colicky pain that radiates into the ipsilateral testicle or labium due to the innervation of the ureter by the genitofemoral nerve. Distal ureteral stones near the ureterovesical junction and stones in the bladder can cause irritative voiding symptoms (urinary frequency, urgency, and dysuria) as well as suprapubic pain. In some cases, pain can radiate to the tip of the penis or to the labia.

Patients often have gross or microscopic hematuria. Some patients will describe passing tea-colored urine. Most patients will have at least microhematuria. However, 10% to 15% of patients with microscopic or gross hematuria ureteral obstruction may present without hematuria. Nonspecific symptoms of urinary stone disease may include nausea and vomiting. Fever and chills often indicate an infection or obstruction in the upper urinary tract, or both.

■ Diagnostic Evaluation

Laboratory Findings

Urinalysis usually shows hematuria, unless complete obstruction prevents urine drainage from the affected side. Urine microscopy is important and can often detect the specific stone morphology and type. Calcium oxalate stone crystals are envelope shaped, whereas cystine crystals tend to be hexagonal. Pyuria may also be present if the stone is associated with urinary tract infection. Urine pH above 7.2 suggests the possibility of a MAP stone, whereas a pH below 5.5 may suggest a uric acid stone. Serum creatinine level may be elevated, especially in the setting of bilateral ureteral obstruction or obstruction in a solitary kidney. Mild leukocytosis (10,000 to 15,000/mm^2) is common because of a stress response; however, white counts greater than 15,000/mm^2 suggest significant infection or urinary tract obstruction or both.

Imaging Studies

A plain film of the kidney, ureters, and bladder (KUB) is usually ordered first in the workup of calculi disease because 80% to 90% of all urinary calculi are radiopaque. Calcium stones are radiopaque and can be seen on plain film as dense, irregularly shaped calcifications (Figure 2-1). In contrast, phleboliths, which

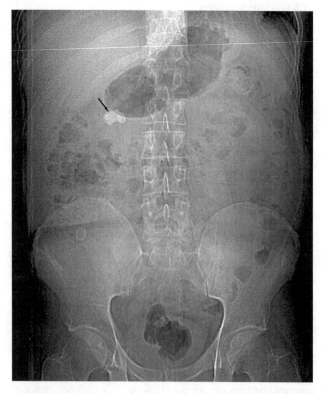

Figure 2-1 • Urolithiasis. KUB film demonstrates a large right renal calcification. *(Used with permission of Cedars-Sinai Medical Center, Los Angeles, California.)*

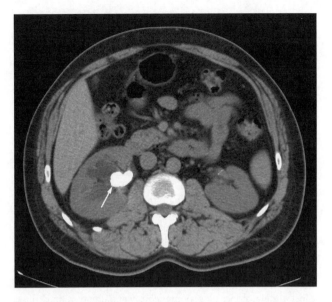

Figure 2-2 • Urolithiasis. Computed tomographic scan of the same patient in Figure 2-1, with right renal collecting system calculus.

are calcifications in the pelvic veins, are well circumscribed but can be confused with calcium stones.

Noncontrast helical computed tomography (CT) is the imaging study of choice. In addition to the presence of the stone, a CT scan helps rule out other potential abdominal pathology. Although the diagnostic yield of a CT scan approaches 100%, the composition of the stone cannot be determined, since all stones appear radiopaque on CT scan. Sometimes, urinary calculi can be confused with calcifications in the pelvic veins known as phleboliths. The presence of a soft tissue swelling (soft tissue rim sign) around the calculus and streaking of the perinephric fat around the kidney further suggests the presence of a urinary tract calculi. These signs are not usually found in association with phleboliths (Figure 2-2).

For patients who are not allergic to administration of intravenous contrast, intravenous pyelography (IVP) may also be used as a first-line test. Stones may appear as filling defects. However, one must also consider that the presence of a filling defect can also represent a blood clot or an upper tract transitional cell carcinoma (TCC). In patients who are at risk for TCC, further evaluation with retrograde pyelography and cytology may be necessary. Other findings on IVP that suggest urinary tract stone disease include the presence of hydronephrosis, delayed excretion of contrast, or dilation of the ureter with visualization of contrast to the level of the obstructing stone (columnization).

Renal ultrasound is useful in patients who are pregnant, those with renal insufficiency, or patients with contrast allergy. This test is operator dependent, with an average sensitivity of 92% and a specificity of 83%. Small stones less than 5 mm are difficult to visualize with ultrasound. Stones may appear as a hyperechoic area with or without associated hydronephrosis. The combination of ultrasound and KUB film may be as effective as IVP in establishing a diagnosis of urinary tract calculi.

Retrograde pyelography is typically not used as an initial test to determine the presence of renal calculi. It may be used in further delineating upper tract anatomy. The procedure involves diagnostic cystoscopy to evaluate the bladder and the placement of a small ureteral catheter into the ureter. Radiographic contrast is instilled in a retrograde fashion, and intermittent fluoroscopic images are taken to further illustrate the anatomy of the upper urinary tract.

■ Treatment

Most ureteral stones pass spontaneously and do not require intervention. The size and location of the stone are two important factors in planning therapy. Distal ureteral calculi measuring less than 4 mm have a 90% chance of passing spontaneously, as compared with only a 10% to 20% chance for stones larger than 6 mm. This does not mean that a 1-cm stone will not pass or that smaller stones (1–2 cm) will pass with ease. The vast majority of stones that pass do so within a 6-week period after the onset of symptoms. Distal stones have a 50% chance of spontaneous passage, whereas proximal stones have a 10% to 25% chance of passing spontaneously. Stones located in higher portions of the proximal ureter (close to the renal pelvis) have a 10% chance of spontaneous passage.

Pharmacologic

DISSOLUTION THERAPY. Oral alkalization therapy with sodium bicarbonate, potassium bicarbonate, or potassium citrate to maintain a urine pH of 6.5 to 7.0 may dissolve uric acid and cystine stones. Patients can self-monitor urine pH daily using Nitrazine paper. Patients with uric acid stones may also benefit from a low-purine diet, whereas patients with cystine stones benefit from restricting foods high in methionine, such meat and dairy products. Struvite stone dissolution requires acidification of urine to a pH of 4.0 using urease inhibitor agents such as acetohydroxamic acid. In general, a minimum of 4 to 6 weeks is necessary before dissolution therapy is considered a failure. The overall effectiveness of dissolution agents is dependent on stone size, location, stone type, and the volume of irrigant used.

SPECIFIC MEDICAL THERAPY. **Absorptive hypercalciuria type I** and renal hypercalciuria are treated with thiazide diuretics and potassium citrate alkalinization. Thiazide diuretics increase tubular reabsorption of calcium in the distal renal tubule. A starting dose of 25 mg may be titrated based on urinary calcium levels. Sodium cellulose phosphate binds calcium in the gut. It is a popular treatment of absorptive hypercalcuria type I associated with recurrent calcium stone formation. The drug decreases urinary saturation of calcium phosphate and calcium oxalate. **Absorptive hypercalciuria type II** is generally managed through diet modification. Sodium cellulose phosphate and thiazide diuretics can also be used. Enteric hyperoxaluria is treated with calcium supplements.

Allopurinol is used to treat hyperuricosuric calcium nephrolithiasis with or without hyperuricemia. This agent inhibits xanthine oxidase and inhibits conversion of hypoxanthine and xanthine to uric acid. Serum and urine levels of uric acid are reduced. Therapy starts at 300 mg/day. It is tolerated best when taken after meals. The occurrence of a skin rash should prompt immediate discontinuation because of the risk of Stevens-Johnson syndrome.

Thiol derivatives, such as D-penicillamine, and α-mercaptopropionylglycine (α-MPG), will decrease urinary cystine excretion by binding to cystine and forming a soluble complex. Thus, D-penicillamine is used in the treatment of cystine stones. An initial dose of 250 mg/day in three to four divided doses may help to limit side effects. Typical adverse effects include rashes and hematologic, renal, and hepatic abnormalities.

Mercaptopropionylglycine (Thiola) is better tolerated than D-penicillamine and is the preferred treatment of cystine stones. This agent binds to cystine and forms a water-soluble compound (Thiola cysteine). Side effects include drug-induced fever, nausea, vomiting, rash, lupuslike syndrome, altered taste perception, and hematologic disorders.

Surgical Treatment

A stone causing any degree of obstruction associated with signs of infection, such as fever, leukocytosis, or pyuria, requires immediate decompression of the collecting system to reduce the risk of pyonephrosis. Usually, a retrograde ureteral stent is placed in the ureter via the urethra to allow adequate drainage; if a ureteral catheter is unable to bypass the stone, a percutaneous nephrostomy tube may be used. Decompression is important to reduce the risk of pyelovenous, pyelotubular, and pyelosinus backflow of infection, which can cause sepsis. Box 2-1 describes the indications for surgical intervention for urinary tract calculus disease.

■ **BOX 2-1 Indications for Surgical Intervention**

Progressive or high-grade obstruction
Intractable pain
Associated infection
Significant hematuria
Stone growth
Large stone size
Solitary

EXTRACORPOREAL SHOCK-WAVE LITHOTRIPSY. Extracorporeal shock-wave lithotripsy (ESWL) has become an accepted treatment for most renal and ureteral stones. Stone composition and location influences the success of ESWL. Stones need to be relatively radiopaque to allow visualization during fluoroscopy. Calcium oxalate stones respond best to shock-wave therapy, whereas cystine stones are relatively resistant.

ESWL success approaches 90% for renal pelvic and proximal ureteral stones smaller than 2 cm. Stones located in the lower pole of the kidney are associated with a lower success rate because the dependent anatomic position of the lower-pole calyces hinders clearance of stone fragments. The success rates for ESWL are similar to ureteroscopic stone extraction for ureteral stones less than 1.5 cm. However, success rates for renal pelvis stones tend to favor ESWL over ureteroscopic extraction. A ureteral stent is often placed prior to the procedure when the stone burden exceeds 2 cm. This will assist in the drainage of the kidney and may aid in stone passage. Most stone fragments pass within 2 weeks of ESWL. Follow-up imaging studies are recommended to guide additional treatment. In some cases where ESWL is ineffective, ureteroscopic extraction with laser lithotripsy becomes an important treatment option.

Contraindications to ESWL include pregnancy, bleeding diathesis, the presence of a large abdominal aortic aneurysm, body habitus (gross skeletal abnormalities, contractures, weight greater than 300 lb), and renal failure. Individuals with cardiac pacemakers require evaluation by a cardiologist prior to ESWL and may need to have the pacemaker overridden during the ESWL procedure.

PERCUTANEOUS NEPHROSTOLITHOTOMY. The percutaneous, antegrade endoscopic approach is the treatment of choice for large stones (>2.5 cm), staghorn calculi, those resistant to ESWL, select lower-pole calyceal stones, or stones in a kidney with ureteropelvic junction obstruction. Percutaneous nephrostolithotomy (PCNL) involves percutaneous passage of an endoscope directly into the collecting system of the kidney through a small flank incision. Needle puncture is directed by fluoroscopy, ultrasound, or both, and is routinely into a posterior inferior or middle calyx. Complications include bleeding and access-related injuries to adjacent structures such as colon and spleen.

URETEROSCOPY. Ureteroscopy is highly efficacious for distal ureteral calculi. Ureteroscopy involves a retrograde endoscopic approach using a small-caliber ureteroscope. Various graspers, baskets, and fragmentation devices, such as holmium or candela laser lithotripsy fibers, can be placed through the ureteroscope. Success rates for distal ureteral stones range from 66% to 100% and are dependent on the stone burden, location, length of time the stone has been impacted, history of retroperitoneal surgery, and the experience of the surgeon. Postoperative complications range from 5% to 30% and include ureteral stricture, ureteral perforation, bleeding, and vesicoureteral reflux.

OPEN SURGERY. Open surgery for removal of urinary calculi is infrequently used because of the advancement of endoscopic equipment and technology. Pyelolithotomy is effective for large stones in an extrarenal pelvis. Anatrophic nephrolithotomy is used for complex staghorn calculi. Ureterolithotomy may be an option for long-standing ureteral calculi that are inaccessible with endoscopy or those that are resistant to ESWL.

ACQUIRED OBSTRUCTIVE UROPATHY

Retroperitoneal Fibrosis (Ormond's Disease)

Retroperitoneal fibrosis (RPF) is a chronic inflammatory process with formation of fibrous plaques centered near the lower lumbar vertebrae.

■ Epidemiology

RPF is relatively uncommon, with a prevalence of 1 in 200,000. It is usually diagnosed between the ages of 40 and 60. The male-to-female ratio is 2:1.

■ Pathogenesis

RPF appears as thick, woody-hard plaques engulfing the retroperitoneal structures. The ureters are the first structures to be functionally compromised. Recent evidence suggests that RPF is an immunologic response to the leakage of an insoluble lipid (ceroid) from thinned arterial walls of an atherosclerotic blood vessel.

■ Risk Factors

In two-thirds of patients, no etiologic factor is found. In the remaining one-third, the most common risk factor is medication use, including prolonged methysergide therapy for migraine headaches. Other implicated causes include inflammatory bowel disease, sclerosing cholangitis, collagen vascular disease, abdominal aortic aneurysm, postirradiation therapy, and chemotherapy.

■ Clinical Manifestations

The symptoms are nonspecific and often include low back pain, malaise, anorexia, and weight loss. Uremia can result from long-standing renal compromise. The diagnosis is made by classic findings that include medial deviation of the ureters with proximal dilation on excretory urography and hydronephrosis. CT scan may show a symmetric, geometrically shaped dense mass anterior to the sacral promontory. A biopsy of the mass is important to rule out malignant disease.

■ Treatment

Idiopathic RPF may respond to corticosteroids or immunosuppressive therapy or both. Agents such as azathioprine, cyclophosphamide, and tamoxifen are often used. Placement of ureteral stents or percutaneous nephrostomy tubes may be necessary in the setting of acute obstruction. Definitive surgery is the preferred treatment when there is poor response to corticosteroids or if the disease process is advanced.

Benign Prostatic Hyperplasia

Benign prostatic hyperplasia (BPH) is a benign progressive enlargement of the prostate seen most commonly in older men. The clinical symptoms of bladder outlet obstruction (BOO) are most likely due to the combination of a mass-related increase in urethral resistance and an obstruction-induced detrusor dysfunction. BOO can lead to urinary tract infection and bladder calculi secondary to urinary stasis from incomplete bladder emptying. Untreated obstruction can also lead to bladder wall changes, detrusor hypertrophy, and atrophy of renal parenchyma due to increased back-pressure from urinary retention.

■ Epidemiology

Histologic evidence of BPH is seen in 40% of men aged 50 to 60 and up to 80% of men aged 70 to 80. The clinical prevalence of BPH increases from 25% of males at 50 to 40% after age 70. At age 55, approximately 25% of men report obstructive voiding symptoms. At age 75, 50% of men complain of decrease in the force and caliber of their urine stream.

■ Pathogenesis

The etiology of BPH remains unclear, but seems to be multifactorial and endocrine controlled. Prostate is composed of both stromal and epithelial tissues, and its growth is under the influence of testosterone and its more potent metabolite dihydrotestosterone (DHT). Testosterone is converted to DHT in the prostate cell by the enzyme 5-alpha reductase (5AR). Growth of BPH involves a balance between cell proliferation and apoptosis. Androgens both enhance cell growth and decrease apoptosis. The mechanical obstruction of the prostatic urethra caused by the hypertrophied tissue is referred to as the **static component** of BPH.

Estrogens have also been implicated in the development of BPH by increasing the number of DHT receptors, which subsequently increases DHT formation.

The **dynamic component** of obstruction refers to the resistance contributed by the tone of the prostatic smooth muscle. Smooth muscle is present in hyperplastic stromal nodules, the bladder neck, and the prostatic capsule. The contractile properties of prostatic smooth muscle are mediated primarily by α_1-adrenergic receptors. Certain patients might report worsening of symptoms in response to increased levels of stress, change in temperature, or certain foods.

BPH is a progressive disease, with ongoing obstruction, bladder wall thickening, and trabeculation; diverticula can develop as a compensation to outflow obstruction. Hydroureter and hydronephrosis may also result from sustained high-pressure bladder storage and sustained high intravesical voiding pressures.

■ Risk Factors

Risk factors for the development of BPH are poorly understood. Some studies have suggested a genetic predisposition, and some have suggested racial differences. Nearly 50% of men who undergo BPH-related surgery and are younger than 60 may have a heritable form of the disease.

The only positive correlations for risk factors are increasing age and normal androgen status. Some data suggest that first-degree relatives of patients with early-onset BPH have four times the risk for development of BPH.

■ Clinical Manifestations

Signs and Symptoms

Obstructive symptoms include hesitancy, small-caliber weak stream, straining to void, incomplete bladder emptying, and terminal and

■ TABLE 2-1 Symptoms of Benign Prostatic Hyperplasia	
Obstructive Symptoms	**Irritative Symptoms**
Hesitancy	Urgency
Weak stream	Frequency
Straining to void	Nocturia
Incomplete bladder emptying	Urge incontinence
Terminal dribbling	
Postvoiding dribbling	

postvoid dribbling. Patients may also complain of irritative symptoms such as urgency, frequency, nocturia, and urge incontinence. These symptoms are commonly referred to as lower urinary tract symptoms (LUTS). Table 2-1 lists the typical BPH symptoms.

■ Diagnostic Evaluation

The self-administered questionnaire developed by the American Urologic Association (AUA) is both valid and reliable in identifying the need to treat patients and is useful in monitoring the response to therapy. The questionnaire is composed of seven items that quantify the severity of the patient's irritative and obstructive voiding symptoms on a scale of 0 to 5. The questionnaire is administered on the first patient visit and again at follow-up evaluations. The score can range from 0 to 37. A symptom score of 0 to 7 is considered mild, 8 to 19 is considered moderate, and 20 to 35 is considered severe. Approximately 80%, 15%, and 5% of patients have mild, moderate, and severe scores, respectively.

Digital rectal exam (DRE) is important to determine the size, shape, symmetry, and consistency of the prostate. Any suspicious areas should be biopsied. The size of the prostate on DRE does not correlate with symptom severity or degree of urodynamic obstruction. A palpable or percussible bladder suggests a retained urine volume of greater than 150 mL in adults.

Laboratory Evaluation

Urinalysis and culture are necessary to rule out a urinary tract infection. An increased serum creatinine level is an indication for upper urinary tract imaging to rule out hydronephrosis. Patients with renal insufficiency are at increased risk to develop postoperative complications after surgical intervention for BPH.

A prostate-specific antigen (PSA) level is a necessary screening test to rule out malignancy, especially when DRE is abnormal. PSA may be falsely elevated in the presence of infection or after a prostate biopsy. A DRE does not significantly affect serum PSA levels.

Special Studies

Cystoscopy allows for direct visualization and estimation of the degree of prostatic enlargement. Cystoscopy is optional in the workup for BPH, but is essential when ruling out other causes of outlet obstruction, such as bladder cancer. Other indications for cystoscopy include a history of risk factors for urethral stricture, microscopic or gross hematuria, and when surgical intervention is considered.

Uroflowmetry is commonly used as a noninvasive tool to measure urine flow rate. Normal peak flow rates are greater than 20 mL/s, and values less than 15 mL/s are indicative of urinary stream impairment. Uroflowmetry cannot differentiate between obstruction and decreased bladder contractility or between the different causes of obstruction.

Postvoiding residual (PVR) is obtained using a portable ultrasound scanner or by direct bladder catheterization after voiding (straight cath). A normal PVR is less than 50 mL. A high PVR does not predict bladder or renal damage or an increased risk of infections or bladder calculi. However, the increased PVR suggests a difficulty with bladder emptying either due to bladder hypocontractility, bladder outlet obstruction, or a combination of both factors.

■ Treatment

Although BPH is a progressive disease, some patients do undergo spontaneous improvement or resolution of their voiding symptoms. Therefore, mild voiding symptoms can usually be observed over time. However, those with moderate or severe symptoms typically need some form of therapy. Indications for treatment include chronic urinary infections, urinary retention, bladder calculi, hydroureteronephrosis, and renal failure. An algorithm for the treatment of BPH is shown in Figure 2-3.

Pharmacologic

PHYTOTHERAPY. **Phytotherapy** refers to the use of plants and plant extracts for medicinal purposes. Plant extracts such as saw palmetto, African pygeum, and *Hypoxis rooperi* have been used by patients in Europe for years, and their use in the United States is growing as a result of patient-driven enthusiasm. The mechanism of action of these phytotherapies are unknown, and the efficacy and safety of these agents have not been tested in randomized clinical trials.

α-ADRENERGIC ANTAGONISTS. The bladder neck, prostatic stroma, and prostate capsule are richly innervated with α_{1a} receptors that control smooth muscle contraction. Selective alpha blockers, such as

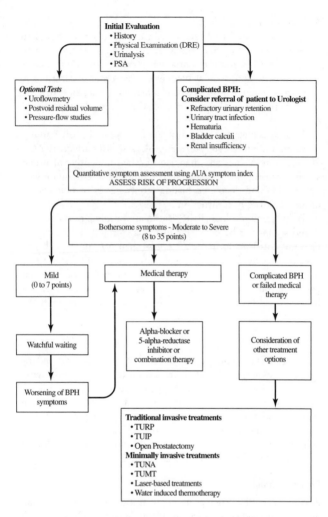

Figure 2-3 • Treatment algorithm for benign prostatic hyperplasia.

terazosin (Hytrin) and doxazosin (Cardura), relax the muscles in the prostate and thus may relieve symptoms. These long-acting alpha blockers are dosed in a daily fashion but require dose titration. Tamsulosin (Flomax) is a more selective alpha blocker that does not require dose titration to achieve success and is associated with a lower risk of potential side effects. It has become a leading choice for the treatment of BPH. Potential side effects of the alpha blockers include orthostatic hypotension, dizziness, and nasal stuffiness.

Several randomized, double-blind, placebo-controlled trials comparing terazosin, doxazosin, and tamsulosin with placebo have demonstrated an improvement in AUA symptom score and urinary flow rate with the alpha blockers.

5-ALPHA REDUCTASE INHIBITORS. 5-alpha reductase (5AR) inhibitors block the conversion of serum testosterone to the more biologically active dihydrotestosterone. As a result, finasteride (Proscar) or dutasteride (Avodart) can induce the shrinkage of the prostate by 25% within 3 months, as well as a 50% decrease in PSA levels. The best results with 5AR inhibitors are seen with large prostates (>40 g). Recent studies suggest the use of 5AR inhibitors in patients with obstructive symptoms that do not respond to alpha blockers and whose PSA is greater than 1.5 mg/mL. Reports also indicate an improvement in AUA symptom score and urinary flow rate after the medications have been used for about 2 to 3 months. A recent report suggests that 5AR inhibitors may decrease the rate of urinary retention and the need for BPH-related surgery in men with enlarged prostates and moderate to severe urinary symptoms. A current study is evaluating the role of 5AR inhibitors in the prevention of prostate cancer. Adverse effects of 5AR inhibitors include decreased libido, decreased ejaculate volume, impotence, and hair growth.

Surgical

TRANSURETHRAL INCISION OF PROSTATE. Transurethral incision of prostate (TUIP) is most efficacious in patients with small prostates (<30 g), especially when bladder neck hyperplasia is present. This procedure involves incising the prostatic urethra and bladder neck with a cutting electrode to reduce urethral resistance. Outcomes are similar to that achieved with transurethral resection of the prostate, although a lower rate of retrograde ejaculation (25%) has been reported with TUIP.

TRANSURETHRAL RESECTION OF PROSTATE. Transurethral resection of prostate (TURP) is an endoscopic procedure in which a resectoscope is placed transurethrally and the obstructing lobes of the prostate are removed as chips of tissue. Approximately 95% of prostatectomies for BPH can be done in this fashion. The remainder are done as open prostatectomies, usually because of larger gland size. TURP results in improvement of flow rate, and symptom scores are superior to that of other minimally invasive therapies. However, the rates of morbidity and mortality associated with TURP are higher.

The risks of TURP include retrograde ejaculation (75%), impotence (5%–10%) and incontinence (<1%). Complications include bleeding, urethral stricture, bladder neck contracture, and perforation of the prostate capsule. A severe complication of TURP is associated with intravascular volume expansion when hypotonic irrigants used during the procedure are absorbed through the prostatic venous plexus. This results in transurethral resection (TUR) syndrome. TUR syndrome is characterized by hyponatremia, mental confusion, nausea, vomiting, and hypertension. The risk of TUR syndrome increases with resection times over 90 minutes. The treatment for TUR syndrome includes diuresis and may require administration of hypertonic saline solution.

TRANSURETHRAL NEEDLE ABLATION. Transurethral needle ablation (TUNA) of the prostate is performed by placing interstitial radiofrequency needles through the urethra and into the lateral lobes of the prostate, causing heat-induced coagulation necrosis. TUNA results in short-term improvement in urinary flow rate and symptom scores. However, comparative long-term randomized studies are lacking.

TRANSURETHRAL MICROWAVE THERAPY. Transurethral microwave therapy (TUMT) involves the insertion of a specially designed urinary catheter into the bladder, allowing a microwave antenna to be properly positioned within the prostatic fossa. This mode of therapy uses microwaves to create heat for destruction of hyperplastic prostate tissue. TUMT results in short-term improvement in urinary flow rate and symptom scores. However, comparative long-term randomized studies are lacking.

SIMPLE PROSTATECTOMY. A simple prostatectomy is performed in patients with very large glands (>80 mL volume). Open prostatectomy is also indicated for patients with a concomitant bladder diverticulum or when a bladder stone is present. Through either a suprapubic or retropubic approach, the hyperplastic tissue located within the transition zone is removed. This mode of therapy results in modest improvements in urinary flow rate, voided volumes, and symptom scores. Only a urethral drainage catheter is needed after the procedure. Risks include impotence, incontinence, retrograde ejaculation, and bladder neck contracture.

Urethral Stricture

Urethral stricture is a narrowing of the urethral lumen secondary to fibrosis or scar formation that results from injury or inflammation to the urethra. Acquired strictures are common in men but rare in women.

■ Pathogenesis

Urethral strictures are most often due to trauma, infection, instrumentation of the urethra, or congenital factors. Straddle injuries and motor vehicle accidents associated with pelvic fractures can cause strictures in the bulbar or membranous urethra. Sexually transmitted diseases (STDs) such as gonococcal urethritis were the most common cause, but the incidence has decreased with effective antibiotic treatment. Infection related to the presence of an indwelling urinary catheter is also a common cause. Larger catheters can be associated with urethral ischemia, which predisposes to stricture. It is important to rule out urethral carcinoma.

The stricture is actually a fibrotic narrowing of the urethra that is composed of dense collagen and fibroblasts. The narrowing causes a restriction of urine flow and dilation of the urethra proximal to the defect. Prostatitis and bladder muscle hypertrophy are sequelae of chronic urethral stricture disease. Vesicoureteral reflux, hydronephrosis, renal failure, urethral fistula, and periurethral abscess can also occur with chronic, severe stricture disease.

■ Risk Factors

Any activity that portends a high risk of acquiring sexually transmitted diseases, such as multiple partners or unprotected sex, may lead to infection, inflammation, and the possibility of fibrosis and stricture formation. Chronic catheterization, as seen in patients with neurogenic bladders, causes repeated trauma to the urethra.

■ Clinical Manifestations

Signs and Symptoms

Patients often complain of lower urinary tract symptoms consistent with obstructive voiding. Symptoms include dysuria, weak stream, incomplete emptying, and postvoiding dribbling. Strictures of the urethral meatus result in deviation or splitting of urinary stream.

■ Diagnostic Evaluation

Retrograde urethrography (RUG) can provide information about the location, length, and caliber of stricture. Sonography has also been a useful method to evaluate urethral stricture disease. Urethroscopy allows direct visualization of the stricture and confirms urethrography findings. Urethral fistulae, diverticula, stones, and bladder trabeculations may be identified.

■ Treatment

Short-term management includes urethral dilation with filiforms or urethral sounds or both, although this is associated with a high

recurrence rate. Optical internal urethrotomy (OIU) utilizes ure-
throtome cutting or electrocautery to ablate the stricture under
direct visualization. OIU has excellent short-term results with
slightly better long-term results compared with urethral dilation.
Open urethroplasty is usually reserved for strictures that fail conservative therapy or for patients with moderate to severe strictures measuring greater than 2.0 cm.

■ Complications and Prognosis

Urinary tract infection, periurethral fistulae, and abscesses can
occur that require antimicrobial therapy or surgical repair or both.
A stricture should not be considered cured until it has been observed for at least 1 year after treatment. Recurrence rates are
highest within the first year after treatment. Patients are followed
periodically with measurement of urinary flow rate, residual volume, and urethrograms.

3

Sexual Dysfunction

MALE SEXUAL DYSFUNCTION

Physiology of Sexual Function

To achieve penile erection, four physiologic events are needed: intact neuronal innervation, intact arterial supply, corporal smooth muscle relaxation, and intact veno-occlusive mechanics.

Visual stimuli and desire are processed in the thalamus, and messages are relayed via the autonomic thoracolumbar and sacral centers to the external genitalia. Afferent fibers of the pudendal nerve carry tactile and sensory stimuli from the penis to the sacral dorsal horn and induce a parasympathetic reflex via the S2–S4 nerve roots that is carried by the cavernous and dorsal nerves to the genitalia. Stimulation of the nerve endings causes release of various neurotransmitters, such as prostaglandins and nitric oxide (NO). NO is released from the endothelial cells, which causes trabecular smooth muscle relaxation via stimulation of guanylate cyclase and production of cyclic guanosine monophosphate (GMP). Cyclic GMP is an important intracellular messenger and is metabolized to GMP by the enzyme phosphodiesterase. These neurotransmitters cause relaxation of the smooth muscle of cavernosal arteries. As erectile tissue of the penis fills with blood, the emissary veins collapse, and venous outflow is obstructed. This causes the penile corpora to become engorged, increasing their length and girth and resulting in erection.

Emission refers to release of secretions from the periurethral glands, seminal vesicles, and prostate. Sperm from the ampulla of the vas deferens are deposited into the posterior urethra as a result of the rhythmic contraction of smooth muscle. Emission is under sympathetic control from the presacral and hypogastric nerves that originate at the T10–L2 cord levels.

Ejaculation involves closure of the bladder neck, which prevents retrograde flow and opening of the external urethral sphincter. Closure of the bladder neck and the contractions of the striated muscles are under sympathetic control (T10–L2). The result is an antegrade flow of ejaculate fluid from the anterior urethra, resulting in completion of orgasm.

Following orgasm, detumescence takes place. A refractory period in which a full erection cannot be achieved ensues.

Erectile Dysfunction

Erectile dysfunction (ED) is defined as the inability to initiate or sustain a penile erection sufficiently to permit penetration for sexual intercourse. Penile erections involve an integration of complex physiologic processes involving the central nervous system (CNS), peripheral nervous system, and hormonal and vascular systems. Any abnormality involving these systems, whether from medication or disease, has a significant impact on the ability to develop and sustain an erection, ejaculate, and experience orgasm.

Four other conditions are important to consider with regard to erectile dysfunction. **Premature ejaculation** refers to persistent ejaculation with minimal stimulation or before the person wishes it. **Retarded ejaculation** is a delay in reaching climax during sexual activity. **Retrograde ejaculation** implies backflow of semen into the bladder after ejaculation secondary to incomplete contraction of the bladder neck during the ejaculatory process. **Anorgasmia** is the inability to achieve an orgasm during sexual activity.

■ Epidemiology

The Massachusetts Male Aging Society found that 52% of men 40 to 70 years of age have some degree of ED. Complete ED affects 5% of men at age 40 years and 25% of men at age 65 years. The National Health and Social Life Survey of men aged 18 to 59 revealed that other male sexual dysfunctions are prevalent in addition to ED. Premature ejaculation (29%), lack of sexual interest (16%), anxiety about sexual performance (17%), and lack of pleasure in sex (8%) are important entities to be considered by physicians who are counseling patients with ED.

■ Risk Factors

Medical risk factors associated with erectile dysfunction include hypertension, hypercholesterolemia, diabetes, cigarette smoking, alcoholism, atherosclerosis, neurologic disorders, and peripheral vascular disease. Diabetes mellitus is a very important risk factor because 50% of such patients have erectile dysfunction. The disease affects small vessels as well as the cavernosal smooth muscle and endothelial cell function.

■ **Pathogenesis**

ED may occur from one or more of the three common mechanisms: failure to initiate (neurogenic or psychogenic), failure to fill (arteriogenic), or failure to store (veno-occlusive).

Vasculogenic causes that result in decreased pelvic blood flow include atherosclerosis, diabetes mellitus, and Leriche's syndrome (impotence secondary to aorto-iliac thromboembolic occlusion). In addition, postpriapism fibrotic changes may result in diminished erections. Venogenic causes (venous leakage) due to the failure of corporal occlusion may also be implicated.

Neurogenic impotence is classified into central and peripheral lesions. Peripheral lesions, such as diabetic neuropathy, are commonly found. Other causes that involve the peripheral autonomic nerves are spinal cord injuries, multiple sclerosis, cauda equina lesions, and tabes dorsalis. Central nervous system diseases causing ED include Parkinson's disease and Huntington's chorea.

Disruptions of the hypothalamic-pituitary-testes axis, including genetic abnormalities, result in ED. Androgens, such as testosterone, are necessary to maintain adequate libido and erectile and ejaculatory functions. The most common endocrine dysfunction associated with ED is hypergonadotropic hypogonadism, as seen in Klinefelter's syndrome. Examples of congenital hypogonadotropic hypogonadism are Prader-Willi and Kallmann's syndromes.

Psychotropic drugs, specifically the selective serotonin reuptake inhibitors (SSRIs) and common antihypertensive agents (alpha and beta blockers), are prevalent and often reversible causes leading to ED.

Once thought to be primarily a psychogenic disorder, ED is now known to be primarily organic in nature (90% of cases). Alcohol, barbiturates, cocaine, and marijuana abuse are also common causes (Table 3-1).

■ TABLE 3-1 Causes of Erectile Dysfunction	
Type	**Causes**
Neurogenic	Diabetes mellitus, tabes dorsalis, multiple sclerosis, spinal cord injury, poliomyelitis, postoperative pelvic surgery
Vascular	Atherosclerosis, diabetes mellitus, Leriche's syndrome, priapism, thrombosis
Endocrine	Primary and secondary hypogonadism, Klinefelter's syndrome, panhypopituitarism, end-stage liver disease
Drug induced	Alcohol, antihypertensive drugs, psychotropic drugs (antidepressant, antipsychotic), barbiturates, cimetidine
Psychogenic	Stress, performance anxiety, depression

■ Clinical Manifestations

History

Organic impotence has an insidious onset, whereas psychogenic impotence often arises suddenly. In addition, if the patient describes waking up in the morning with an erection (nocturnal penile tumescence), a psychogenic etiology is very likely. Obtaining a social history is important in assessing recent stressors, especially psychosocial issues such as marital discord or loss of employment.

■ Diagnostic Evaluation

In addition to a complete physical examination, some focus should also be placed on assessing the vascular (peripheral pulses), neurologic (radiculopathy, lumbosacral reflexes), and endocrinologic (secondary sexual characteristics) aspects.

The use of a self-report measure is important to assess male sexual function. The Sexual Health Inventory for Men (SHIM) is a five-item questionnaire that assesses the domains of sexual function, including erectile function, orgasmic function, sexual desire, intercourse satisfaction, and overall satisfaction. Each area is given a score of 1 to 5, where 5 represents no problem in the area and 1 represents significant difficulty in the area. ED severity is then classified into five categories: severe ED (score of 5–7), moderate ED (8–11), mild to moderate ED (12–16), mild ED (17–21), and no ED (22–25).

Laboratory Studies

Routine workup should be performed to include basic laboratory tests such as a complete blood count, urinalysis, fasting blood glucose level, serum creatinine level, lipid profile, and morning serum testosterone and prolactin levels.

Special Studies

Duplex ultrasonography is a vascular diagnostic test that consists of an intracavernosal injection and measurement of blood flow by duplex Doppler ultrasound. This test is the most reliable and least invasive evidence-based assessment of ED. Ultrasound can detect the peak systolic velocity through the cavernosal arteries and the diastolic flow after the injection. In normal subjects, there is an increase in arterial flow through the cavernosal artery (>30 cm/s) and absence of diastolic flow (venous leakage). Ultrasound is also useful to uncover penile abnormalities such as Peyronie's plaques, thickened vessel walls, and fibrosis of the corporal bodies.

Nocturnal penile tumescence and rigidity (NPRT) testing measures nocturnal erection frequency, rigidity, and duration. A normal man has three to four erections during the night, each lasting for 20 to 30 minutes during rapid eye movement (REM) sleep. This test is useful in differentiating psychogenic from neurogenic impotence.

Cavernosometry measures the intracavernosal pressures while saline flow rates needed to obtain and maintain full erection are determined. **Cavernosography** is useful for patients with partial erections, in whom venous leakage is suspected. Contrast is infused into the corpora cavernosa, and radiographic imaging is performed to document venous leakage.

Other vascular testing, such as **internal pudendal angiography**, is reserved for patients who have a recent history of pelvic trauma, where precise location of arterial injury is necessary. In addition, it is used for patients with a history of arterial occlusion who are candidates for penile artery bypass surgery.

■ Treatment

PHOSPHODIESTERASE INHIBITORS. **Sildenafil (Viagra)** is a potent, selective inhibitor of type V phosphodiesterase, resulting in increased levels of cyclic guanosine monophosphate (cGMP). Sexual stimulation and intact nerve conduction is necessary. Overall, 57% to 85% of men with ED achieve a satisfactory response with Viagra. As far as specific etiologies are concerned, Viagra is effective in 70% of patients with hypertension, 57% of diabetic patients, 43% of patients after radical prostatectomy, and 80% of patients after spinal cord injury. Side effects include headaches (15%), facial flushing (11%), nasal congestion (4%), and transient vision disturbances (3%). It is contraindicated in patients on nitrate therapy because it can precipitate a hypotensive response.

Vardenafil (Levitra) is a newly released, possibly more potent, and selective inhibitor of type V phosphodiesterase than sildenafil. Preliminary data suggest that this agent may show as much promise as sildenafil in the management of erectile dysfunction. Phase II trials at doses of 2.5, 5, 10, or 20 mg showed success rates of completed intercourse between 71% and 75% after 8 to 12 weeks of treatment. The most commonly reported adverse effects were headache, flushing, and rhinitis.

Tadalafil (Cialis) is another newly released phosphodiesterase inhibitor. Tadalafil is a highly potent and selective inhibitor of type phosphodiesterase V. In phase II trials, the percentages of successful intercourse attempts were 46%, 62%, 70%, and 70% for tadalafil doses of 5, 10, and 20 mg, respectively. This agent has a long half life (17.5 hours) which can provide for erections up to 36 hours after taking this pill. This may result in improved efficacy and patient satisfaction. The most common adverse effects were headache, dyspepsia, and myalgias.

Apomorphine is a dopamine receptor agonist that activates D1 and D2 receptors. Dopamine stimulation can produce an erection. A sublingual form of dopamine is approved in Europe for the treatment of ED. This product has not received approval from the Food and Drug Administration (FDA) in the United States. Studies suggest that 2-mg and 4-mg doses produce erections satisfactory for intercourse in 43% and 55% of patients, respectively. Adverse effects include nausea (17%), dizziness (8%), sweating (5%), yawning (8%), and sleepiness (6%).

Yohimbine is a centrally acting α_2-adrenergic antagonist derived from tree bark. Clinical studies have shown only moderate success, although it seems to be effective in psychogenic impotence. Side effects include palpitations, headache, agitation, anxiety, and increases in blood pressure.

INTRACAVERNOSAL INJECTION THERAPY. Prostaglandin E_1 (PGE_1, alprostadil) is available as an intracorporeal injection or as a urethral pellet. PGE_1 works by increasing cAMP concentration in the cavernosal smooth muscle by providing substrate for adenylate cyclase. Dosages are titrated to achieve an erection lasting 30 to 60 minutes. At therapeutic doses, alprostadil injection produces full erection in 70% to 80% of patients with ED. The most frequent side effects are pain at the injection site during erection (17%), hematoma (2%), and prolonged erection (2%). The percentage of patients who accept injection therapy ranges from 50% to 85%; however, approximately 13% to 60% will drop out over time. The most common reasons for dropout include penile pain, inadequate response, fear of needles, lack of a partner, and loss of sex drive.

VACUUM ERECTION DEVICE. Mechanical treatment involves the use of a vacuum erection device or pump along with a constriction ring. The penis is placed in a vacuum tube and the air is pumped out, creating a negative pressure to allow blood flow to the penis. This noninvasive mode of therapy is effective in treating erectile problems from most causes, although the device can be cumbersome to use. Complications include penile pain, numbness, difficulty with ejaculation, ecchymosis, and petechiae. The initial patient satisfaction rate ranges from 53% to 83%. However, a significant number of patients drop out over time for reasons similar to those described for intracavernosal injection therapy.

TESTOSTERONE REPLACEMENT THERAPY. Testosterone replacement therapy is used for improving ED in cases of primary testicular failure or hypogonadotropic hypogonadism. Testosterone replacement is available via intramuscular injection or transdermal formulations. Testosterone is contraindicated in patients with a history of prostate cancer or symptomatic benign prostatic hyperplasia

(BPH). In addition, relative contraindications include significant coronary artery disease and hyperlipidemia, because testosterone can increase serum triglyceride levels. Elevated prolactin levels require a complete endocrinologic workup.

Surgical Treatment

PENILE PROSTHESIS. Penile prostheses are divided into three types: malleable (semirigid), mechanical, and inflatable devices. These devices are appropriate for patients who have failed therapy with oral agents or those who have a severe arterial or venous cause of impotence. They are also appropriate for patients with neuropathic impotence. Patient and partner satisfaction with this form of therapy are 85% and 80%, respectively. There is a 5% to 15% device failure rate for the first 5 years after implantation. Most patients will need revision surgery by 10 to 15 years. Potential complications of penile implants include mechanical failure, cylinder and tubing leaks, infection, perforation, and autoinflation.

PENILE VASCULAR SURGERY. Isolated pudendal arterial disease in young patients after pelvic trauma may be revascularized with penile vascular surgical procedures. The most commonly used technique is a bypass from the inferior epigastric artery to the dorsal artery or the deep dorsal vein of the penis.

Related Topics

Premature Ejaculation
Premature ejaculation is defined as a recurrent or persistent ejaculation with minimal stimulation before, during, or shortly after the vagina is entered. There is usually an underlying psychological disorder. Psychotherapy involving behavioral modification using the "squeeze technique" described originally by Masters and Johnson is approximately 90% effective. Pharmacotherapy includes application of topical anesthetics and use of SSRIs.

Retrograde Ejaculation
Retrograde ejaculation occurs when impairment of the muscles or nerves of the bladder neck prohibit it from closing during ejaculation, allowing semen to flow backward into the bladder. The condition of the bladder neck may be a result of bladder neck surgery, a developmental defect in the urethra or bladder, a disease that affects the nervous system (e.g., diabetes), or be associated with the use of alpha blockers in the treatment of BPH. Therapeutic trials of medications to induce bladder neck closure have been suggested for this condition. Agents such as pseudoephedrine, phenylephrine, and antihistamines have been tried with reasonable success.

Peyronie's Disease
....

Peyronie's disease (PD) is a sexually disabling condition characterized by a fibrotic scarring and plaque formation of the tunica
albuginea and corpora cavernosa of the penis.

■ Epidemiology

PD predominantly occurs in men aged 40 to 60 years. The incidence is 0.3% to 4.0% among white men and is less common in
men of African American or Asian heritage.

■ Pathogenesis

The exact etiology of PD remains unclear, although microtrau-
matic events are implicated in the pathogenesis. Trauma causes
collagen and fibrin to accumulate in the form of a plaque, generally along the dorsal and ventral midline aspects of the penile
shaft. PD may also be associated with erectile dysfunction, diabetes mellitus, hypertension, and use of beta blockers. Among
patients with PD, 10% have Dupuytren's contracture, while 3%
of patients with Dupuytren's contracture have PD.

■ Diagnostic Evaluation

Signs and Symptoms
Initially, patients complain of painful erections, but are usually
asymptomatic in the flaccid state. Gradually, curvature of the
penis progresses, sometimes until penetration and intercourse are
difficult. Decreased sensation and diminished erection distal to
the plaque may also be present. A palpable fibrous plaque may
be evident on physical examination.

Laboratory and Radiographic Findings
Features of the history and the physical examination findings are
usually adequate to make the correct diagnosis. High-resolution
ultrasonography is the definitive imaging study, although it is not
required to confirm the diagnosis. Ultrasonography may be helpful before definitive surgical intervention is planned. Duplex
Doppler ultrasonography may reveal arterial, venous, or combined diseases suggesting an underlying erectile dysfunction.

■ Treatment

Mild cases usually require no treatment because 50% of the cases
often regress, provided that the patient is able to have intercourse
comfortably. If remission does not occur, various medical treatments exist with limited success. Treatment with potassium *p*-
aminobenzoate (POTABA) is effective in reducing pain and

improving deformity. Other treatments include oral vitamin E supplementation, intralesional steroids, and calcium channel blocker therapy. The most effective treatment is surgical excision of the plaque with grafting, plication, and/or implantation of a penile prosthesis. Indications for surgery are impotence or severe deformity of the penis that prevents sexual intercourse.

Priapism

Priapism is a prolonged and painful erection that is not associated with sexual thoughts or sexual activity. This process affects only the corpora cavernosa, while the corpora spongiosum of the glans penis and surrounding the urethra remains flaccid. Detailed information about this condition is provided in Chapter 11.

FEMALE SEXUAL DYSFUNCTION

Female sexual dysfunction (FSD) is a multicausal and multidimensional medical problem that has biological and psychosocial components. Etiologic factors include chronic medical conditions (diabetes, hypertension, hypercholesterolemia), minor ailments (arthritis), medications, and psychosocial difficulties, including prior physical or sexual abuse. The diagnosis of FSD requires obtaining a detailed patient history that defines the dysfunction, identifies causative or confounding medical and gynecologic conditions, and elicits psychosocial information.

Female Sexual Response and Physiology of Sexual Arousal

The female sexual response cycle consists of four stages of arousal, marked by physiologic and psychological changes. The first stage is **excitement,** which can be triggered by psychological or physical stimulation and is characterized by emotional changes, increased heart rate and respirations, and vaginal swelling and lubrication due to increased blood flow to the iliohypogastric pudendal arterial bed with simultaneous relaxation of the vaginal wall smooth muscle. Engorgement within the vaginal wall increases pressure within the blood vessels, enabling a process of plasma transudate formation to occur.

The second stage is the **plateau.** Vaginal swelling, heart rate, and muscle tension may increase as long as stimulation continues. The breasts enlarge, the nipples become erect, and the uterus dips in position.

The third stage is **orgasm,** which involves synchronized vaginal, anal, and abdominal muscle contractions, the loss of involuntary muscle control, and intense pleasure.

The final phase, **resolution,** involves a rush of blood away from the vagina, shrinking breasts and nipples, and a reduction in heart rate, respiration, and blood pressure.

Hormone levels in the body affect female sexual function. Estrogens have a vasodilatory effect that increases vaginal, clitoral, and urethral arterial flow through the regulation of the expression of nitric oxide synthase (NOS), the enzyme responsible for the production of nitric oxide. In addition, estrogen is important in the function and thickness of vaginal epithelium, as well as vaginal lubrication. Age-related decline in estrogen results in vaginal wall atrophy and dryness. This may ultimately result in complaints of female sexual dysfunction such as dyspareunia.

Decreased sexual arousal, libido, sexual responsiveness, genital sensation, and orgasm can also be associated with low levels of testosterone. Studies show that menopausal women respond better to parenteral estrogen–androgen combinations than to estrogen alone with regard to enhanced sexual desire, libido, energy, sexual motivation, and overall sense of well-being.

■ Epidemiology

Female sexual dysfunction is an age-related and progressive problem estimated to affect 30% to 50% of women. Most female sexual dysfunction occurs during or after menopause, when hormone production drops and vascular conditions are more common. Higher prevalence of sexual dysfunction is observed in women who have had negative sexual experiences such as forced sex or adult–child sexual contact.

Diagnostic Classification of FSD

Female sexual dysfunction can be subdivided into disorders of sexual desire, sexual arousal, orgasm, and sexual pain.

■ Sexual Desire Disorders

Hypoactive Sexual Desire Disorder
Hypoactive sexual desire disorder is defined as the persistent deficiency or absence of sexual fantasies and thoughts and of receptivity to sexual activity, which causes personal distress. This condition may result from psychological factors or may be secondary to physiologic problems, such as hormone deficiencies and medical or surgical interventions that decrease hormone levels.

Sexual Aversion Disorder

Sexual aversion disorder is the persistent avoidance of sexual contact with a partner, which causes personal distress. This condition is generally a psychological or emotional-based problem that can result from a variety of causes, such as physical or sexual abuse or childhood trauma.

Sexual Arousal Disorder

Sexual arousal disorder is the persistent or recurrent inability to attain or maintain sufficient sexual excitement, causing personal distress. Disorders of arousal include lack of or diminished vaginal lubrication, decreased clitoral and labial sensation, decreased clitoral and labial engorgement, and lack of vaginal smooth muscle relaxation. Most commonly, these conditions are secondary to a disruption in the normal sexual physiologic response, such as diminished vaginal or clitoral blood flow, prior pelvic trauma, pelvic surgery, or medications.

Orgasmic Disorder

Orgasmic disorder, classified as primary or secondary, is the persistent or recurrent difficulty in, delay in, or absence of attaining orgasm after sufficient sexual stimulation and arousal, which causes personal distress. In addition to hormonal deficiencies, primary anorgasmia may result from emotional trauma or sexual abuse.

■ Sexual Pain Disorders

Dyspareunia

Dyspareunia is recurrent or persistent genital pain associated with sexual intercourse. In addition to having a psychogenic origin, dyspareunia can develop secondary to medical problems such as endometriosis, vaginal atrophy, or vaginitis.

Vaginismus

Vaginismus is the involuntary contraction of the perineal muscles around the lower third of the vagina, primarily the levator ani, in response to attempted penetration. Contraction makes vaginal penetration difficult or impossible. Vaginismus usually develops as a conditioned response to painful penetration or develops secondary to psychological or emotional factors.

Noncoital Sexual Pain Disorder

Other sexual pain disorders cause recurrent or persistent genital pain induced by noncoital sexual stimulation.

■ Pathogenesis

Lack of female sexual arousal has been associated with medical conditions similar to those described for male impotence, such as hypertension, hypercholesterolemia, smoking, and heart disease. All these conditions predispose patients to acquiring atherosclerotic disease, which causes a diminished pelvic blood flow that results in vaginal wall atrophy, dryness, and dyspareunia. In addition, injuries to the pelvic vasculature can result in symptomatic diminished vaginal blood flow and complaints of sexual dysfunction. Such injuries can result from pelvic fractures, blunt trauma, surgical disruption, or chronic perineal pressure from bicycle riding.

Hypothalamic-pituitary axis dysfunction, menopause, premature ovarian failure, and long-term contraceptive use are the most common causes of hormonal- and endocrine-related female sexual dysfunction. Sexual dysfunction can also result from central or peripheral neuropathies such as spinal cord injuries or diabetes, which can impair genital sensitivity. Orgasmic dysfunctions occur when there are no motor or sensory functions in the genital organs, including the pelvic floor muscles.

Emotional, self-esteem, body image, and relational issues can significantly affect sexual arousal. In addition, depression and anxiety disorders are associated with female sexual dysfunction. Medications used in treating depression such as monoamine oxidase inhibitors and, more commonly, selective serotonin reuptake inhibitors (SSRIs) have been associated with decreased desire, decreased arousal, decreased genital sensation, and difficulty achieving orgasm. In addition, psychotropic agents, certain pain medications, and illicit drug abuse have been implicated in causing sexual dysfunction.

■ Diagnostic Evaluation

Signs and Symptoms

Patients often present with complaints of decreased desire and libido, vaginal dryness, lack of sexual arousal, inability to reach an orgasm with adequate sexual stimulation, and painful sexual intercourse. Patients may also complain of vaginal burning, itching, irritation, pressure, or urinary problems.

A detailed patient history that defines the dysfunction, identifies causative or confounding medical or gynecologic conditions, and elicits psychosocial information is important prior to physical examination.

The use of patient questionnaires is helpful in further quantifying the dysfunction. The Female Sexual Function Index (FSFI) is a 19-item questionnaire that classifies FSD into disorders in six domains: desire, arousal, orgasm, satisfaction, lubrication, and pain.

■ BOX 3-1 Differential Diagnosis of Painful Intercourse in Women

Vaginal atrophy
Bartholin's gland cyst
Urethritis
Persistent hymen
Vaginitis
Endometriosis
Cystitis
Iatrogenic stenosis after surgery or childbirth
Retroverted uterus
Postinflammatory or postsurgical adhesions

This questionnaire provides initial diagnostic information and can be useful at follow-up visits to assess response to treatment.

Evaluation should include a thorough physical examination, including a pelvic examination, which may recreate the pain symptoms. The differential diagnosis of common conditions that cause painful intercourse is provided in Box 3-1.

Laboratory Evaluation

As with evaluation of the male patient with ED, basic laboratory studies to identify underlying conditions may be important. Thus, routine urinalysis, urine culture, complete blood count and liver function tests, and serum cholesterol and glucose levels are important to obtain. Specialized laboratory testing should be guided by patient symptoms and examination findings. The suggested hormonal profile includes assays for follicle-stimulating hormone (FSH), luteinizing hormone (LH), prolactin, total and free testosterone levels, sex hormone-binding globulin (SHBG), and estradiol levels.

In patients in whom vaginitis, cervical cancer, or a sexually transmitted disease is suspected, cultures and vaginal samples should be obtained first. Vaginal pH testing via probe may assist in detecting bacteria-causing vaginitis. Decreasing hormone levels and diminished vaginal secretion associated with menopause cause a rise in pH (>5), which is easily detected with the test.

Imaging Studies

Vaginal blood flow and engorgement can be objectively measured with **vaginal photoplethysmography,** in which an acrylic tampon-shaped instrument inserted in the vagina uses reflected light to sense flow and temperature. Genitosensory analysis is another evolving experimental diagnostic test of FSD.

■ **Treatment**

Hormone replacement therapy (HRT) is aimed at restoring hormone levels affected by age, surgery, or hormone dysfunction to normal, thus restoring sexual function. In addition to relieving symptoms of hot flashes, and slowing osteoporosis, HRT increases clitoral sensitivity, increases libido, and decreases pain and burning during intercourse. Topical estrogen creams relieve symptoms of vaginal dryness, burning, and urinary frequency and urgency.

Topical testosterone cream is currently used in treating vaginal lichen planus. Potential benefits of this therapy include increased clitoral sensitivity, increased vaginal lubrication, increased libido, and heightened arousal. All androgens carry the risk of developing hirsutism and clitoromegaly, and eventually of inducing virilization in women.

Sildenafil (Viagra), used in men with erectile dysfunction, is currently being tested in women. Some evidence suggests that it may improve sexual functioning in women who are taking an SSRI. Viagra is also being evaluated in women after radical hysterectomy in an effort to determine if clitoral and vaginal blood flow are increased as well as sensitivity.

In addition to the medical treatments, all patients should be evaluated and treated for emotional or relational issues that may contribute to the several dysfunctions.

Male Infertility

Hypothalamic-Pituitary-Gonadal Axis

The hypothalamic-pituitary-gonadal axis plays a vital role in normal testosterone production and spermatogenesis. Gonadotropin-releasing hormone (GnRH) is released from the medial basal hypothalamus in a pulsatile pattern approximately every 70 to 90 minutes. It travels down the portal system to the anterior pituitary, where it stimulates the release of luteinizing hormone (LH) and follicle-stimulating hormone (FSH). After release into the systemic circulation, FSH and LH exert their effect by binding to plasma membrane receptors of the target cells in the testes. LH mainly functions to stimulate testosterone secretion from the Leydig cells of the testicle (steroidogenesis), whereas FSH stimulates Sertoli cells to facilitate germ cell differentiation (spermatogenesis). Gonadotropin release is regulated through negative feedback by a variety of hormones, such as estradiol (a potent inhibitor of both LH and FSH release), and inhibin from the Sertoli cell, which causes a selective decrease in FSH release (Figure 4-1).

Prolactin, also a hormone secreted from the anterior pituitary, inhibits the pulsatile secretion of GnRH from the hypothalamus and of LH and FSH from the pituitary. Men with elevated prolactin levels present with gynecomastia, decreased libido, erectile dysfunction, and galactorrhea.

Male Infertility

Infertility is the inability of a couple to conceive after 1 year of unprotected sexual intercourse.

■ Epidemiology

Over 4.5 million men and women in the United States, approximately one in five couples, fail to conceive during their first attempt at pregnancy. A male factor for infertility can be identified in 30% to 40% of cases and is a contributing factor in 50% of cases.

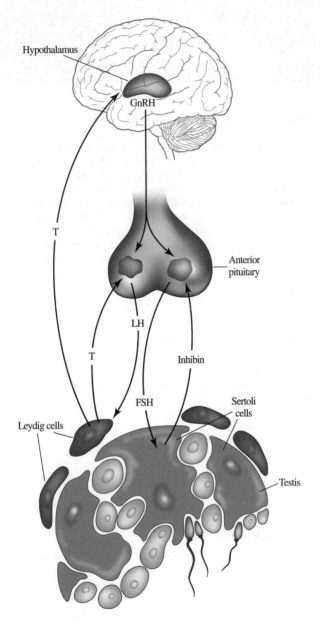

Figure 4-1 • Hypothalamic-pituitary-gonadal axis. GnRH (gonadotrophin releasing hormone); T (testosterone); LH (leutenizing hormone); FSH (follicle stimulating hormone).

■ Pathogenesis

The etiology of male infertility can be categorized into pretesticular, testicular, or post-testicular causes, all of which eventually lead to problems with sperm production or delivery. Certain environmental factors have been demonstrated to have an effect on infertility. For example, cigarette smoking and marijuana use lead to decreased libido, sperm density, and motility, and abnormal sperm morphology. Alcohol has been shown to produce both an acute and a chronic decrease in testosterone secretion. Excessive heat exposure from saunas, hot tubs, or the work environment may cause a temporary decrease in sperm production.

Pretesticular causes of infertility include congenital or acquired diseases of the hypothalamus, pituitary, or peripheral organs that result in an alteration of the hypothalamic-pituitary axis. The disorders of the hypothalamus that lead to **hypogonadotropic hypogonadism** result in the lack of GnRH secretion; therefore, no pituitary gland secretion of LH and FSH can occur. This phenomenon is seen in Kallmann's syndrome (midline defects such as anosmia, deafness, and cryptorchidism), Prader-Willi syndrome (obesity, mental retardation, and micropenis), and Laurence-Moon-Biedl syndrome (retinitis pigmentosa and polydactyly).

Testicular causes can be divided into chromosomal and nonchromosomal causes. Klinefelter's syndrome (47,XXY) is the most common chromosomal cause of male infertility and is characterized by a eunuchoid body, gynecomastia, and small testes. Other less common causes are XYY and XX karyotypes and Noonan's syndrome (webbed neck and short stature). Most of these syndromes are associated with primary testicular failure, manifesting as decreased levels of testosterone and increased gonadotropins (FSH, LH, prolactin).

Varicocele is an example of a nonchromosomal testicular cause of infertility; it is the most common cause of male infertility. A left-sided varicocele is found in 15% of healthy men, and in nearly 40% of all infertile men. Bilateral varicoceles are uncommon in healthy men (<10%), but are palpated in up to 20% of subfertile men. Venous congestion and an unfavorable local environment for spermatogenesis secondary to higher testicular temperature are believed to contribute to oligospermia.

Testicular trauma can cause an abnormal immune response and testicular atrophy following injury. Both of these can contribute to infertility. Trauma usually results in fracture of the tunica albuginea layer of the testicle. When such a fracture is identified by physical or radiologic examination, it should be repaired.

Orchitis is an inflammation of the testicular tissue and is caused by either bacterial or viral infection. Viral infection is common with mumps, and orchitis is observed in 30% of males who have mumps parotitis. Orchitis can lead to formation of antisperm antibodies and development of testicular atrophy.

Testicular torsion can lead to ischemic injury to the testicle. When diagnosed within the first 6 hours, the testicle can usually be saved. However, the torsion can result in release of antisperm antibodies and predispose to male infertility.

Cryptorchidism (undescended testis) is found in 0.8% of boys at 1 year of age. It is considered a developmental defect and places the testis at higher risk of infertility and developing cancer. Prophylactic orchiopexy is generally performed by 2 years of age to allow the testis to be palpated for cancer detection. It is unclear whether orchiopexy alters the fertility potential of patients with undescended testicles.

Post-testicular causes of infertility are due to impaired sperm transportation secondary to congenital or acquired ductal obstruction. Ductal obstruction is caused by repeated infection, inflammation, or developmental defect. Infertility and recurrent respiratory infections may be due to **immotile cilia syndrome.** Immotile cilia may manifest as an isolated disease or as part of **Kartagener's syndrome** with situs inversus and bronchiectasis. Cystic fibrosis is associated with congenital bilateral absence of the vas deferens (CBAVD), leading to obstructive azoospermia. Although both copies of this recessive gene are necessary for clinical disease, the presence of only one copy may lead to CBAVD. Acquired causes usually are secondary to sexually transmitted diseases, such as chlamydia and gonorrhea, but may also include reactivated tuberculosis or smallpox. Table 4-1 presents the differential diagnosis of male infertility in terms of causes that are treatable, potentially treatable, or untreatable.

■ TABLE 4-1 Causes of Male Infertility		
Treatable Causes	Potentially Treatable Causes	Untreatable Causes
Varicocele	Idiopathic	Bilateral anorchia
Ejaculatory dysfunction	Congenital absence of the vas deferens	Primary testicular failure
Phimosis	Cryptorchidism	Bilateral testicular torsion
Hypospadias	Medication use	Infection (mumps, tuberculosis)
Hyperprolactinemia	Surgery/trauma to vas deferens	Chronic liver or renal disease
Antisperm antibodies	Occupational/recreational	Chemotherapy/radiation

■ Clinical Manifestations

History and Physical Examination

Libido, erection, penetration, and ejaculation abilities, in addition to the duration, frequency, and timing of unprotected intercourse, must be noted. Previous pregnancies indicate that the infertility is acquired. A past history of genitourinary infections such as mumps, syphilis, gonorrhea, or chlamydia is relevant. Social history is important to investigate use of cigarettes, illicit drugs, alcohol, and exposure to chemical toxins at the workplace.

Physical examination should be undertaken first in a general sense to inspect for signs of feminization, eunuchoid body habitus, poor muscle development, and lack of secondary sexual characteristics. Examination of the testes should uncover signs of testicular atrophy or swelling. Swelling with pain is indicative of orchitis, whereas nontender enlargement may be observed in testicular neoplasms, tuberculosis, and tertiary syphilis. An enlarged, indurated epididymis with a cystic component should alert the physician to the possibility of ductal obstruction, whereas tenderness may be due to epididymitis. The presence of both vasa deferentia should be noted. A rectal examination should assess the prostate and seminal vesicles.

Laboratory Testing

SEMEN ANALYSIS. A semen analysis (from at least two occasions) is required regardless of what previous tests have shown. Six sperm factors are analyzed in a semen analysis. (Normal values are listed in Table 4-2.) **Azoospermia** is the absence of sperm in the semen, whereas **oligospermia** refers to a sperm count that is lower than 20 million. **Motility** refers to the percentage of sperm moving and is the single most important measure of semen quality. **Asthenospermia** refers to low sperm motility or low forward progression. Forward progression is a quantitative assessment of

■ TABLE 4-2 Normal Semen Parameters	
Parameter	Value
Volume	1.5–5 mL
Sperm density	>20 million/mL
Motility	>60%
Forward progression	>2.0 (scale 0–4.0)
Abnormal forms	<40%
No significant pyospermia, hyperviscosity, or agglutination	

the quality of sperm movement in a forward direction and is graded on a scale from 0 (no movement) to 4.0 (excellent straight-forward movement). Abnormal sperm morphology characteristics include head defects, tail defects, and immature forms.

ANTISPERM ANTIBODIES. Patients with antisperm antibodies usually have a history of testicular trauma, torsion, or infection, where the blood–testes barrier is altered, allowing for an autoimmune reaction against sperm antigen. Semen analysis is usually normal in these patients. An immunobead test assay is used to test for IgG and IgA antibodies. Antisperm antibodies are also commonly seen in postvasectomy patients.

HORMONAL STUDIES. Plasma levels of FSH, LH, testosterone, and prolactin should be measured in all infertile patients. Primary testicular failure is characterized by small testes, azoospermia, and an elevated FSH level. Low gonadotropin levels (LH and FSH) suggest hypopituitarism. An elevated prolactin level should raise the suspicion of a pituitary adenoma, and a full endocrinologic evaluation is necessary.

Imaging Studies
Transrectal ultrasonography (TRUS) helps to identify ejaculatory duct obstruction secondary to prostatic calculi. Dilatation of the seminal vesicles or ejaculatory ducts is seen on TRUS.

Special Studies
Testicular biopsy is useful in azoospermic patients to differentiate between obstructive and nonobstructive azoospermia. In patients with normal-sized testes, normal FSH, and spermatogenesis on testicular biopsy, **vasography** allows accurate localization of the obstruction. Most patients with obstructive azoospermia have an obstruction in the epididymis caused by scarring from previous infection.

■ Treatment

Initial treatment should begin with education on cessation of smoking and drugs, and on modification of alcohol consumption. Occasionally, a couple needs education on the optimal time for sexual intercourse. Intercourse should occur no more than every 2 to 3 days in correlation with ovulation.

Medical Treatment
Antibiotics, such as the quinolones (levofloxacin and ciprofloxacin), are used to treat fertility-impairing infections of the urinary tract, including sexually transmitted diseases (STDs) and chronic prostatitis. Hypogonadotropic states are treated with gonadotropin replacement with human chorionic gonadotropin (hCG)

titrated to restore LH and FSH to normal levels. Hyperprolactinemia secondary to pituitary microadenomas usually responds to treatment with bromocriptine. Macroadenomas are often surgically treated with transphenoidal resection of the pituitary gland. Corticosteroids, such as prednisolone, can be used against antisperm antibodies by reducing IgG and IgA levels. In men with no identifiable cause of infertility, antiestrogen therapy with clomiphene citrate and tamoxifen has proven to be of some benefit.

Assisted Reproductive Techniques

In patients with testicular biopsies positive for mature sperm, such as those with ductal obstruction, CBAVD, and failed vasectomy reversal, various techniques for sperm retrieval for future **assisted reproductive techniques (ART)** are available. Techniques such as **microepididymal sperm aspiration (MESA)** and **percutaneous epididymal sperm aspiration (PESA)** can be used to retrieve sperm. After retrieval, sperm undergo a washing process that separates sperm from white blood cells and prostaglandins in the semen that may hinder sperm motility.

Sperm retrieved by MESA or PESA are used with **in vitro fertilization (IVF)** and **intracytoplasmic sperm injection (ICSI).** IVF involves combining eggs with sperm in a laboratory, and then transferring the resulting embryos to the uterus. ICSI may be used with immotile sperm during in vitro fertilization. Using a tiny glass needle, one sperm is injected directly into a retrieved mature egg. Fertilization occurs in 50% to 80% of cases, and approximately 30% will result in a live birth.

Gamete intrafallopian transfer (GIFT) is a procedure similar to IVF, in which mature eggs and prepared sperm are combined in a syringe and injected into the fallopian tube using laparoscopy. The average conception rate for this procedure is about 30%.

Varicocele

Varicocele is a dilatation of the veins of the pampiniform plexus within the spermatic cord. It is classified into three grades: palpable with only Valsalva maneuver (grade I), palpable without need of Valsalva maneuver (grade II), or visible on inspection (grade III).

■ Epidemiology

Varicoceles are rarely found in children prior to puberty. A varicocele is found in 15% of males in the general population, but is often found in up to 40% of men presenting with infertility problems. The majority of varicoceles occur on the left side.

■ Pathogenesis

Dilatation of the pampiniform veins is caused by valvular incompetence when the spermatic vein is exposed to high venous pressures. The left-sided predominance is due to the variation in venous drainage of the two testes. Several anatomic features contribute to the predominance of left-sided varicoceles. First, the left spermatic vein is longer than the right. In addition, it drains into the left renal vein at a right angle. In contrast, the right gonadal vein drains *obliquely* into the inferior vena cava, acting as a natural valve. Thus, in the standing man, higher venous pressures can be transmitted to the left scrotal veins and result in retrograde reflux of blood into the pampiniform plexus. Rarely, a varicocele develops as a result of a retroperitoneal tumor or thrombus from renal tumor occlusion of the renal vein, thus inhibiting the drainage of the spermatic vein. Such a varicocele often develops on the right side. Thus, the presence of a right-sided varicocele may prompt further evaluation of the retroperitoneum with appropriate imaging studies such as computed tomographic scan.

■ Diagnostic Evaluation

Signs and Symptoms

In the majority of patients, varicoceles are asymptomatic. Higher-grade varices can ache, typically after prolonged standing or toward the end of the day.

Examination should be conducted in a warm room while the patient is standing to allow the veins to fill up. A Valsalva maneuver may help to distend the pampiniform veins by increasing abdominal pressure. Grades 2 and 3 varicoceles feel like a "bag of worms" located on the superior aspect of the scrotum when the patient is standing and usually reduce when the patient lies down. The testicle on the affected side is often smaller when the varicocele has been present for a long time.

Imaging Studies

Physical examination is usually adequate for varicoceles that are symptomatic. An ultrasound with color Doppler can be used to identify "subclinical" varices. The usefulness of repairing "subclinical" varices is controversial in male subfertility and of limited value in cases of orchalgia. The sudden onset of a varicocele in an older individual requires further abdominal imaging to rule out renal cancer with renal vein invasion.

■ Treatment

Treatment of varicocele is necessary only for subfertility, pain, testicular growth retardation in adolescents, or cosmetic reasons for large varicoceles. There is little benefit in treating a varicocele that is asymptomatic. Various surgical techniques for repair of the varicocele include retroperitoneal, inguinal, and subinguinal approaches, laparoscopic clipping, and transvenous embolization. Pain relief is often immediate after surgery, whereas an improvement in semen analysis may take up to 6 months. Recurrence rates have been reported to be as high as 20%, depending on the surgical approach.

Vasectomy

Vasectomy is a safe and effective means of sterilization and an alternative for men seeking birth control. Typically, the procedure is offered to an individual who has a stable marriage and does not desire any further children. Vasectomy is typically performed in an office setting under local anesthesia. The vas deferens is interrupted so that sperm can no longer exit during an ejaculation. Conventional vasectomy is performed through an incision made in the scrotum. The vas is then identified, tied with sutures or blocked with permanent clips, cut, and cauterized. Complications of the procedure include bleeding and subsequent scrotal hematoma, wound infection, and chronic scrotal pain. Patients need to be counseled that a vasectomy is meant to be irreversible, that sperm may appear in the ejaculate for up to 3 months after vasectomy, and that the possibility of recanalization still exists after the procedure.

Vasovasotomy (vasectomy reversal) is an option for men who wish to be fertile again after a previous vasectomy. The success rate varies from 40% to 70% and is higher if the vasectomy was performed less than 5 years prior to the reversal.

Neurogenic Bladder and Voiding Dysfunction

Physiology of Voiding

The bladder has two main functions: to store urine at a low pressure and to expel urine in a coordinated, controlled fashion. This coordinated activity is regulated by the central and peripheral nervous systems. The micturition cycle is initiated in the brainstem, specifically, in the **pontine micturition center (PMC)**. This area is controlled by impulses from the **micturition control center (MCC)** located in the frontal lobe of the cerebral cortex, which sends inhibitory signals to the detrusor muscle to prevent the bladder from contracting. This is a trained reflex that helps to prevent the bladder from emptying at an undesirable place and time. In infants, the inhibitory reflex from the MCC is underdeveloped, and the detrusor acts in an uninhibited manner. Stimulation of the PMC is responsible for the coordination of bladder contraction and external sphincter relaxation. Lesions above the T7 region of the spinal cord result in **detrusor-striated sphincter dyssynergia.** In this condition, the external sphincter contracts during voiding instead of relaxing. The detrusor attempts to overcome this pressure by generating higher pressures to void. These pressures are not only transmitted to the external urethral sphincter but also to the upper urinary tract. Thus, such patients are predisposed to hydronephrosis and renal stones and renal infections.

The sympathetic innervation to the bladder is derived from T10 to L2 (hypogastric nerve) and is active during urine storage and compliance. There is little sympathetic innervation of the detrusor muscle. In contrast, sympathetic innervation predominates in the base of the bladder, the internal urethral sphincter, the prostate, and the proximal urethra, via activation of α-adrenoceptors. Parasympathetic nerves from S2 to S4 via the pelvic splanchnic nerve primarily supply the detrusor muscle and are active during micturition. Contraction of the detrusor muscle is mediated primarily by stimulation of muscarinic receptors by acetylcholine.

The urethral sphincter has both striated and smooth muscle components. The internal sphincter is an involuntary smooth muscle sphincter innervated primarily by the sympathetic component (hypogastric nerve). Conversely, the external sphincter is a voluntary striated muscle sphincter that receives its motor supply from somatic nerves (pudendal nerves) derived from the sacral region. Sensory nerve fibers that detect the degree of stretch in the bladder wall, fullness, and pain are also carried by the pelvic nerve. These signals are mainly responsible for initiating the micturition reflex.

Neurogenic Bladder

Many neurologic disorders are associated with a disturbance in the normal function of the bladder. Neurologic dysfunction can be categorized into upper motor neuron or lower motor neuron lesions. An **upper motor neuron** (UMN) lesion is a defect between the brain and the anterior horn cells of the spinal cord above the sacral micturition center (S2–S4). **Lower motor neuron** (LMN) lesions are characterized by a defect from the anterior horn cells of the spinal cord to the peripheral organ of innervation. These LMN lesions include damage from spinal trauma to the sacral region, pelvic surgery, and diabetes mellitus. Lesions at any point in the neurologic pathway can disturb the continence and voiding mechanism. It is important to remember that because the neurologic control of the bladder is complex, no two lesions will result in the same clinical symptoms.

Upper Motor Lesions

■ Cerebral Disorders

Neurologic lesions above the PMC usually result in involuntary bladder contractions because of the loss of inhibitory function of the cerebral cortex. This also affects the voluntary function of cortical inhibition, leading to detrusor overactivity. Because the PMC is not affected, external sphincter synergy is maintained. In addition, sensation and voluntary external sphincter control are intact. Therefore, patients often complain of frequency, urgency, incomplete voiding, and incontinence due to **detrusor hyperreflexia**. Common conditions that present in this fashion include cerebrovascular accident, Parkinson's disease, and cerebral tumors.

■ Spinal Cord Injuries

Spinal shock is a period of time following spinal cord injury during which there is decreased excitability at and below the affected spinal segment. This leads to **detrusor areflexia**, a paralysis of the detrusor that results in retention of urine. The bladder and sphincter start to regain reflex activity as they recover from spinal shock. It takes between 2 and 12 weeks to recover from spinal shock.

In contrast to cerebral lesions, spinal cord injuries occur below the PMC and above the T7 spinal level, resulting in **detrusor sphincter dyssynergia with detrusor hyperreflexia (DSD-DH)**. The patient will demonstrate symptoms of urinary frequency, urgency, and urge incontinence but will not be able to empty the bladder completely. This occurs because the urinary bladder and the sphincter are overactive and contract simultaneously. Therefore, high bladder pressures are needed to overcome sphincter pressures. As mentioned previously, this may eventually result in detrusor hypertrophy, ureteral reflux or obstruction, hydronephrosis, and renal impairment.

Lower Motor Neuron Lesions

Injury to the sacral cord most commonly results in detrusor areflexia, resulting in urinary retention. Urinary incontinence usually does not occur because the bladder still maintains compliance. Characteristically, the bladder capacity is large, intravesical pressure is low, and involuntary contractions are absent. Because smooth muscle is intrinsically active, fine trabeculations in the bladder may be seen.

Diabetes mellitus results in a neuropathy involving the autonomic nerves to the bladder that causes sensory and motor deficits. Loss of sensation allows for overstretching of the detrusor, with delays in the desire to void. Eventually, this may progress to chronic retention of urine with overflow incontinence and recurrent urinary tract infections.

■ Clinical Manifestations

Neuropathic bladder disorders may present with a variety of signs and symptoms. It is necessary to elicit a proper history of the onset and duration of the symptoms, history of trauma, medical conditions (diabetes mellitus, strokes, multiple sclerosis), and medications that might affect bladder function (particularly psychotropic and anticholinergic agents). Patients may also complain of changes in bowel habits or erectile dysfunction or both, which may indicate sacral nerve dysfunction. Detrusor hyperreflexia may cause urinary frequency, urgency, or urge incontinence. An areflexic bladder or a bladder with detrusor-sphincter dyssynergia may be associated with complaints of urinary hesitancy, poor urinary stream, and overflow incontinence. Chronic urinary retention in these patients may lead to chronic urinary tract infections, renal and bladder calculi, and chronic renal failure.

A physical examination that includes a focused neurologic examination is important, because symptoms of a neurogenic bladder may mimic other causes of lower urinary tract symptoms. The abdomen should be palpated for masses. A digital rectal examination (DRE) in males is necessary to access the size of the prostate to exclude benign prostatic hypertrophy, which may also cause lower urinary tract symptoms. Neurologic examination should include testing for anal sphincter tone, contraction of the pelvic floor muscles, and presence of the bulbocavernosus reflex. This reflex evaluates the integrity of sacral nerves S2–S4. In addition, the presence of intact sensation of the lower extremities and of the perineal and pericoccygeal region, and the presence of deep tendon reflexes and motor strength of the lower extremities should be evaluated.

■ Diagnostic Evaluation

Initial laboratory investigations should include a urinalysis and urine culture to rule out a urinary tract infection, and serum blood urea nitrogen and creatinine levels to assess renal function. In addition, a renal ultrasound should be performed to rule out hydronephrosis or stone disease and assess kidney size. Patients with a history of unremitting low back pain with neurologic deficits should undergo magnetic resonance imaging to examine for lumbar disc disease and spinal or metastatic tumors. Urodynamic studies are the gold standard used to evaluate bladder and urethral function. These studies assess bladder filling (cystometrogram) and emptying (pressure/flow). Neurogenic bladder conditions can have abnormalities in bladder filling, bladder emptying, or both processes.

Incontinence

Urinary incontinence is a *symptom* defined as the involuntary leakage of urine that results in a social or hygienic problem. Incontinence can be demonstrated objectively. Normally, urinary continence is maintained by the dynamic interplay between the urethral sphincter, which is normally closed except during voiding, and the bladder's dynamic ability to fill with large volumes of fluid without significant rises in pressure.

Urinary incontinence has been estimated to occur in approximately 15 million adults in the United States, with the majority affected being female. It is estimated that one in four women experiences incontinence during her lifetime. The incidence increases with age; more than 50% of women in nursing homes suffer from incontinence.

■ Classification

Stress Incontinence
Stress incontinence is the involuntary loss of urine as a result of weakness of the pelvic floor, resulting in descent or hypermobility

of the bladder neck and proximal urethra. It is associated with increases in intra-abdominal pressure, and can occur with laughing, sneezing, coughing, and straining. Normally, the urethral sphincter is well supported by the pelvic musculature and is able to respond to increases in bladder filling pressure. The levator muscle contracts to support the proximal urethra and bladder base; therefore, inefficient contraction will lead to leakage of urine. In addition, estrogen plays an important role in maintaining the submucosal vasculature of the female urethra through a mechanism known as **mucosal coaptation**. The estrogen-sensitive vasculature complex helps to maintain the intraurethral pressure when filled with blood. An associated component of intrinsic sphincter deficiency may also contribute to stress incontinence in some patients. Multiple vaginal deliveries, pelvic surgery, menopause, and urethral trauma are all risk factors in women. In men, stress incontinence is most commonly seen in postradical prostatectomy cases due to damage to the external urethral sphincter.

Urge Incontinence

Urge incontinence is the involuntary loss of urine that is preceded by a sudden and strong desire to void. True urge incontinence is usually the result of detrusor instability during bladder filling with a normal functioning sphincter. Other causes include poor bladder compliance, resulting in small functional bladder capacity, and underlying irritating factors such as urinary tract infections, bladder calculi, and cancer. Associated symptoms include urgency, frequency, and nocturia.

Detrusor instability is defined as a spontaneous bladder contraction during bladder filling that results in an objective increase in bladder pressure while attempting to inhibit micturition. The etiology of the uninhibited bladder contractions is not well understood. When detrusor instability is associated with a neurologic deficit, the term **detrusor hyperreflexia** is used instead.

Total (Continuous) Incontinence

Total urinary incontinence occurs when the urethral sphincter is unable to prevent leakage. This may result from damage to the urethral sphincter or from a urinary fistula between the bladder and the vagina (vesicovaginal fistula), bypassing the sphincter. The most common causes of urinary fistulae are pelvic radiation and pelvic surgery, accounting for over 95% of the cases. In these cases, pelvic examination will usually reveal the fistula opening through the vagina. When a vesicovaginal fistula is identified, one must also consider a concomitant ureterovaginal fistula. Identification of these fistulae requires intravenous pyelogram or retrograde urethrogram or both.

TABLE 5-1 Treatment of Common Voiding Dysfunctions		
Type	Symptoms	Therapy
Stress incontinence	Involuntary loss of urine with laughing, coughing, sneezing, or straining	Kegel exercises: To strengthen pelvic floor muscles Estrogen therapy: Women with atrophic vaginitis may benefit from increasing submucosal coaptation α-Adrenergic agonists: To increase internal urethral pressure Surgery: Urethral/suburethral vaginal wall slings; bladder suspensions; or anterior repair
Detrusor instability (urge incontinence, detrusor hyperreflexia)	Involuntary loss of urine associated with urgency, frequency, and nocturia	Bladder training: Scheduled timed voidings Anticholinergic agents: tolterodine (Detrol), oxybutynin (Ditropan), oxybutynin patch (Oxytrol) Tricyclic antidepressants: Imipramine Desmopressin (DDAVP) Surgery: Bladder augmentation (cystoplasty); partial bladder denervation
Detrusor-sphincter dyssynergia (suprasacral spinal cord lesions)	Incomplete voiding, poor urinary stream, and straining	Intermittent catheterization Sacral nerve stimulation
Areflexic bladder (sacral cord lesions, diabetic neuropathy, overflow incontinence)	Urinary dribbling, straining to void, poor stream, incomplete emptying, and retention of urine Diabetes neuropathy typically presents with loss of sensation to void, and with decreased voiding volume due to detrusor hypotonia	Intermittent catheterization α-Adrenergic receptor blockers: To reduce internal urethral closing pressure Diazepam, dantrolene: To relax external sphincter muscles Cholinomimetic agents (e.g., bethanechol): To increase bladder contractility
Total incontinence	History of painless and continuous loss of urine, with a history of pelvic radiation or pelvic surgery	Broad-spectrum antibiotics Fistula-repair surgery

Overflow Incontinence

Urinary leakage associated with overflow incontinence is the result of an overdistended bladder with an intravesical pressure high enough to overcome the urethral closure pressure. Causes of chronic retention include outlet obstruction from benign prostatic hypertrophy (BPH), detrusor hypocontractility from fecal compaction, diabetic neuropathy, spinal cord injuries, and use of medications such as anticholinergics.

■ Clinical Manifestations

Common presenting symptoms of each type of incontinence are described in Table 5-1. History taking should be guided toward ascertaining the underlying cause of the incontinence. Patient voiding dairies are useful and are an objective method for determining frequency, volume of voided urine, and associated symptoms such as leakage. Physical examination should include a complete pelvic examination in females to identify the presence of a pelvic mass, atrophic vaginitis, organ prolapse (cystocele, rectocele), or fistula. A DRE is important in male patients to identify obstruction caused by BPH. DRE in the female may also be important to further evaluate a rectocele.

Primary management of incontinence includes urinalysis to exclude an infection, a serum creatinine level to determine renal function, and cystourethroscopy to exclude bladder calculi, tumors, and fistulae. Pharmacologic and other therapies are listed in Table 5-1.

6 Genitourinary Tract Infections

Urinary tract infections (UTIs) can have multiple risk factors, including anatomic etiologies, the presence of a foreign body, urinary tract stone disease, and immunologic factors. Table 6-1 describes these risk factors and the common etiologies.

In addition to risk factors, the body has established defense mechanisms aimed at preventing infections. Some of the common urinary tract defense mechanisms are listed in Box 6-1.

UPPER TRACT INFECTIONS

Upper tract infections involve the kidney or the surrounding tissues or both.

Acute Pyelonephritis

Acute pyelonephritis is an acute bacterial infection of the renal parenchyma and collecting system. Most commonly, pathogens

■ TABLE 6-1 Risk Factors and Common Etiologies for Urinary Tract Infections

Risk Factor	Examples
Anatomic anomaly causing obstruction, stasis, or reflux	Prostatic hyperplasia Neurogenic bladder Strictures Vesicoureteral reflux Other congenital urinary tract anomalies
Foreign body	Urinary catheter, stent, nephrostomy tube Instrumentation (cystoscope)
Infected urinary stones	Struvite calculi Secondarily infected calculi
Immunologic or biologic disorders allowing bacterial persistence	Chronic bacterial prostatitis Immunosuppression Pregnancy Renal papillary necrosis End-stage renal disease on hemodialysis

■ **BOX 6-1 Urinary Tract Defense Mechanisms**

Maintenance of urine flow
Bladder emptying
Low pH
Extremes in osmolality
High urea concentration
High organic acid concentration
Prostatitic secretions
Antiadherence factors (uromucoid, Tamm-Horsfall protein)
Immunoglobulins
Phagocytosis

ascend from the bladder via the ureter to the renal pelvis and parenchyma. The second route of infection, hematogenous spread, is associated with other extrarenal infections such as staphylococcal septicemia and tuberculosis. Acute pyelonephritis is characterized by suppurative infection accompanied by fever, flank pain, bacteriuria, and pyuria. Progressive renal scarring is a consequence of repeated attacks of acute pyelonephritis.

■ **Pathogenesis**

The origin of most bacteria causing pyelonephritis is in fecal flora. *Escherichia coli* and other Enterobacteriaceae account for over 90% of infections. Other less common pathogens include *Proteus, Pseudomonas, Klebsiella,* and *Enterococcus.* Certain virulence factors have been identified that enhance bacterial ability to colonize, ascend the urinary tract, and produce disease. Of these factors, the most important is bacterial adherence by pili to the vaginal mucosa and uroepithelium. It has also been found that patients with chronic pyelonephritis have a higher P-fimbriae receptor accessibility on uroepithelial cells.

■ **Diagnosis**

The classic presentation of acute pyelonephritis is fever, flank pain, and lower urinary tract symptoms with bacteriuria. Flank pain is often unilateral but rarely can be bilateral. Upper abdominal pain is unusual, and radiation of pain to the groin is suggestive of a ureteral stone. Fever may be accompanied by rigors and chills. Other nonspecific symptoms may include nausea, vomiting, anorexia, and malaise.

On physical examination, the patient generally appears ill. Flank or costovertebral angle (CVA) tenderness is most commonly unilateral over the involved kidney, although bilateral discomfort may be present. A systolic blood pressure less than 90 mm Hg suggests shock secondary to sepsis or perinephric abscess.

The urinalysis typically reveals pyuria, bacteriuria, and gross or microscopic hematuria. The complete blood count (CBC) reveals leukocytosis with a predominance of neutrophils. The serum creatinine level may be elevated due to the transient renal dysfunction. Urine cultures are diagnostic, and the sensitivity results help to determine the appropriate antibiotic therapy. Obtaining blood cultures is important because bacteremia is present in 33% of patients.

Computed tomographic (CT) scan with contrast helps to define the renal parenchyma and surrounding tissues. Contrast-enhanced CT scan may show wedge-shaped areas of decreased contrast enhancement secondary to decreased perfusion of renal parenchyma due to constriction of arterioles caused by acute bacterial infection.

■ Treatment

Acute pyelonephritis is a serious illness that requires prompt treatment. Empiric therapy should cover gram-negative pathogens and can be adjusted according to culture and sensitivity results. One-drug therapy with a third-generation cephalosporin or fluoroquinolone is usually effective. Aminoglycosides plus ampicillin may be required for compromised hosts with nosocomial infections, primarily *Pseudomonas*. Acute pyelonephritis requires 2 weeks of combined IV and oral antibiotics. If symptoms do not begin to improve within 3 to 5 days, further investigation is needed to rule out obstruction or renal abscess, which may require percutaneous drainage or surgical intervention.

Pyonephrosis

Urinary obstruction in the presence of pyelonephritis may lead to a collection of bacteria, purulent drainage and debris in the collecting system, and subsequent pyonephrosis. In this last situation, patients may deteriorate rapidly and become septic.

Risk factors for developing pyonephrosis include immunosuppression, diabetes, and urinary tract obstruction resulting from stones, tumors, or ureteropelvic junction obstruction. Fungal balls, commonly associated with immunocompromised patients, may obstruct the renal pelvis or the ureter, also resulting in pyonephrosis.

■ Diagnosis

Patients usually present with high fever, chills, and flank pain. Ultrasound is usually sufficient to establish the diagnosis. Findings include a dilated collecting system with dependent echoes suggestive of the accumulation of purulent sediment. CT scan is also helpful in diagnosing and delineating the extent of pyonephrosis. Diagnostic criteria for pyonephrosis on CT scan include increased wall thickness of the renal pelvis greater than or equal to 2 mm, the presence of renal pelvic contents and debris, and parenchymal and perirenal findings, such as perirenal fat stranding.

■ Treatment

In addition to broad-spectrum parenteral antibiotics, drainage via ureteral catheter or via percutaneous nephrostomy tube may be necessary to relieve the obstruction.

Emphysematous Pyelonephritis

Emphysematous pyelonephritis (EPN) is a life-threatening, fulminant, necrotizing upper urinary tract infection associated with gas within the kidney or perinephric space or both. This condition typically occurs in patients who are immunocompromised. Diabetics account for 87% to 97% of patients with EPN. The most frequently associated pathogen is *E. coli*, which is believed to utilize necrotic tissue to ferment glucose and produce carbon dioxide gas.

■ Diagnosis

EPN can be diagnosed when acute pyelonephritis fails to resolve within 3 days of appropriate antibiotic therapy. Gas in the region of the kidney on a plain film of the abdomen is a hallmark finding. Ultrasound findings include strong focal echoes suggesting the presence of intraparenchymal gas. CT scan is the ideal study to identify localized gas and to determine the extent of infection.

■ Treatment

Treatment involves aggressive antibiotic therapy and prompt control of blood glucose levels. Surgical treatment includes drainage procedures to relieve obstruction and prompt nephrectomy in life-threatening situations. The mortality rate is as high as 54%. Patients who portend a worse prognosis with EPN include those with an elevated serum creatinine level, thrombocytopenia, and the presence of a perirenal fluid collection associated with gas in the collecting system.

Renal and Perirenal Abscess

Renal abscess is a collection of purulent material confined to the renal parenchyma. A **perirenal abscess** results from the extension of an acute cortical abscess into the perinephric space confined by Gerota's fascia. When a perinephric abscess ruptures through Gerota's fascia into the pararenal space, the abscess is known as a **paranephric abscess**. Historically, most perirenal abscesses evolve from a hematogenous spread from a skin lesion. Patients at high risk for the development of a perirenal abscess include patients on hemodialysis, diabetics, and intravenous drug abusers.

■ Diagnosis

The most common presenting symptoms include fever, flank pain, abdominal pain, chills, and dysuria. Most symptoms will have been ongoing for approximately 2 weeks prior to diagnosis. A flank mass may be palpable in some patients. Urinalysis often reveals white blood cells, but it can be normal in 25% of patients. Urine cultures are positive in 33%, whereas blood cultures are positive in 50%. Renal abscesses can be diagnosed on CT scan or ultrasound. CT scan may demonstrate an enlarged kidney, thickening of Gerota's fascia, perinephric stranding, and obliteration of the soft tissue planes. Ultrasound may reveal an anechoic mass within or displacing the kidney.

■ Treatment

Empiric broad-spectrum antibiotics (ampicillin or vancomycin in combination with an aminoglycoside or third-generation cephalosporin) are recommended. If the patient does not respond to therapy within 48 hours of initiating treatment, percutaneous drainage under CT or ultrasound guidance should be undertaken. Fluid from percutaneous drainage procedures should be sent for microbiologic evaluation with determination of culture and sensitivity. If the abscess still persists, open surgical drainage or nephrectomy may be indicated.

Chronic Pyelonephritis

Chronic pyelonephritis is induced by recurrent or persistent renal infection. It occurs almost exclusively in patients with urologic anomalies, including urinary tract obstruction, struvite calculi, renal dysplasia, or, most commonly, vesicoureteral reflux (VUR). Infection without reflux is less likely to produce injury, whereas repeated bacterial infections with underlying VUR can cause renal insufficiency. Chronic pyelonephritis is associated with progressive renal scarring, which can lead to end-stage renal disease (ESRD).

■ Diagnosis

Symptoms of chronic pyelonephritis are nonspecific, although patients may report fever, lethargy, nausea and vomiting, and flank pain. Failure to thrive may be an initial complaint in some children. Urinalysis may show pyuria, bacteriuria, and proteinuria if significant renal insufficiency is present. In addition, creatinine and blood urea nitrogen levels may be elevated.

An intravenous pyelogram can reveal small, atrophic kidneys, caliceal dilatation with blunting, and cortical scarring. Ultrasound can also demonstrate these findings. Renal scan may reveal renal scarring. A voiding cystourethrogram (VCUG) should be done if VUR is suspected.

■ Treatment

Medical therapy consists of long-term antibiotic therapy to prevent further renal damage. Surgical therapy of VUR is necessary if bacteruria persists despite prophylactic antibiotic therapy. Nephrectomy is usually necessary in patients with renal atrophy, large stone burden in a nonfunctioning kidney, and renin-mediated hypertension.

Xanthomatous Pyelonephritis

Xanthomatous pyelonephritis (XGP) is a chronic inflammatory disorder of the kidney characterized by a mass originating in the renal parenchyma. The clinical characteristics of XGP include calculi (35% of patients) or obstruction in the urinary tract and subsequent renal damage, anemia, increased sedimentation rate, and hepatic dysfunction (50% of patients). The condition is commonly associated with *Proteus* or *E. coli* infection, but the precise etiology is not known.

The gross appearance of XGP is a mass of yellow tissue with regional necrosis and hemorrhage, superficially resembling that of a renal cell carcinoma, which makes it clinically and radiographically difficult to differentiate XGP from renal cell carcinoma. Therefore, nephrectomy is the standard treatment for XGP for diagnostic and therapeutic reasons.

LOWER TRACT INFECTIONS

Cystitis

Cystitis is classified into two categories: simple and recurrent. Approximately 20% of women will have recurrent infections after their first UTI, although subsequent UTIs can be due to a different pathogen than found initially. Factors that promote infection include glucosuria, pregnancy (which changes urine pH and promotes urinary stasis), obstruction, incomplete bladder emptying, atrophic vaginal mucosa, and frequent sexual intercourse. Obstruction is considered the most important predisposing factor. Causes of recurrent cystitis include inadequate treatment, inadequate duration of treatment, and poor patient compliance.

Pregnant women are not only more susceptible to developing UTIs, due to the anatomic and physiologic changes of pregnancy, but also are more susceptible to the ensuing development of pyelonephritis. Untreated pyelonephritis during pregnancy is associated with a high rate of premature delivery and infant mortality. For this reason, bacteriuria in pregnant women is treated regardless of the presence or absence of symptoms.

■ Pathogenesis

Fecal flora is the principal source of bacterial organisms that cause cystitis. Women are predisposed to cystitis because of a short urethra, which allows bacteria to ascend via a fecal-perineal-urethral route. Cystitis can then ensue. The most common pathogens are *E. coli* (80%) and *Staphylococcus saprophyticus* (15%). Less common pathogens include *Proteus mirabilis* and *Klebsiella pneumoniae*.

■ Diagnosis

Symptoms of frequency, urgency, and dysuria are the hallmarks of acute cystitis. Patients may also complain of low back and suprapubic pain. In simple cystitis, fever and other constitutional symptoms are absent. Urinalysis shows pyuria, bacteriuria, and occasionally hematuria. Urinary dipstick tests are positive for bacterial nitrites and leukocyte esterase. Urine culture is necessary to determine the causative organism(s) and antimicrobial sensitivities.

■ Treatment

First-line treatment for uncomplicated cystitis is a short (3–5 day) course of trimethoprim-sulfamethoxazole (TMP-SMX). However, it is estimated that resistance to TMP-SMX by *E. coli* is 20%.

For this reason, nitrofurantoins and fluoroquinolones have been utilized in treatment of UTIs because they have excellent coverage against uropathogens and decreased resistance.

Prostatitis

Prostatitis is an infection or inflammation of the prostate gland that presents as several syndromes with varying clinical features. Prostatitis is one of the most common urologic diagnoses in men under 50, accounting for over 1 million visits per year, with the chronic and nonbacterial prostatitis variants being the most frequently diagnosed.

The four most common syndromes of prostatitis are acute bacterial prostatitis, chronic bacterial prostatitis, chronic nonbacterial prostatitis/chronic pelvic pain syndrome (CP-CPPS), and granulomatous prostatitis. Individuals with acute and chronic bacterial prostatitis have documented bacterial infections of the prostate. Patients with CP-CPPS have signs of prostatic inflammation but no signs of bacterial infection. Examination of prostatic secretions under the microscope may reveal inflammatory cells. Granulomatous prostatitis is an uncommon form of prostatitis that can result from bacterial, viral, or fungal infection or the use of bacille Calmetle-Guérin (BCG) therapy.

Acute Bacterial Prostatitis

Acute bacterial prostatitis is thought to result from an ascending urethral infection or from reflux of infected urine into the prostatic ducts, or both. *Escherichia coli* is the most common cause of acute bacterial prostatitis. Other etiologic organisms include *Enterobacter, Proteus, Klebsiella,* and *Pseudomonas.* Patients present with acute onset of lower back pain and perineal pain, fever, chills, urinary urgency and frequency, dysuria, and hematuria. Digital rectal examination (DRE) reveals a warm, tender, enlarged, boggy prostate. Prostatic massage and vigorous prostate examination should be avoided, because these can promote bacteremia. Patients with persistent urinary retention secondary to acute prostatitis should be managed with a suprapubic catheter because transurethral catheterization or instrumentation is not recommended.

Physical examination reveals the classic findings mentioned previously. A complete blood count may show leukocytosis. Voided urine often reveals pyuria, microscopic hematuria, and bacteria. Urine culture usually isolates the causative organism.

Either fluoroquinolone or trimethoprim-sulfamethoxazole for 30 days is adequate for treatment and may be important in the prevention of chronic bacterial prostatitis.

Chronic Bacterial Prostatitis

The causative organisms of chronic bacterial prostatitis are the same as those of acute prostatitis. In addition to the intraprostatic reflux described previously, free zinc (known as a prostatic antibacterial factor) is found in low levels in men with chronic bacterial prostatitis. Zinc has been shown to have some bactericidal activity against some gram-negative organisms.

Patients present with milder symptoms compared with those of acute prostatitis, including perineal and low abdominal pain, dysuria, poor stream, pain on ejaculation, and hematospermia. A DRE is usually normal. However, it is not uncommon to have tenderness or firmness of the prostate on DRE.

Fractionated urine specimens remain the hallmark of the diagnosis of chronic bacterial prostatitis. Serial collection of the urine (first voided bladder specimen [VB_1], midstream bladder specimen [VB_2], expressed prostatic secretions [EPS], and residual bladder specimen [VB_3]) is used to define and identify the involved organisms. A positive VB_1 culture indicates urethritis or prostatitis or both. A positive VB_2 culture indicates cystitis. Positive EPS or VB_3 indicate prostate infection. Urine cultures before and after massage of the prostate may also help in the diagnosis. Chronic bacterial prostatitis can be diagnosed if the culture of the prostatic secretions and postmassage urine cultures grow the same bacteria as the first-voided specimen and if the colony count of the two cultures is at least 10 times greater than the first-void specimen.

Choices of antimicrobial agents are similar to that of acute prostatitis, although they are prescribed for at least 6 weeks' duration. Therapy for 12 weeks is recommended.

Chronic Nonbacterial Prostatitis/Chronic Pelvic Pain Syndrome

Nonbacterial prostatitis is an inflammatory condition of unknown etiology with symptoms similar to those of chronic bacterial prostatitis. Some studies have shown that *Chlamydia trachomatis* may play a role. Nonbacterial prostatitis is estimated to be 8 times more frequent than its bacterial counterpart.

Clinical features are similar to those of chronic bacterial prostatitis. Perineal, penile, and testicular pain predominate, and voiding symptoms include dysuria, frequency, urgency, and weak stream. Patients may have symptoms of bladder outlet obstruction and decreased urinary flow rate. Spasms of the bladder neck and external sphincter due to increased adrenergic stimulation may cause intraprostatic reflux of urine. DRE may reveal an increased sphincter tone and tender paraprostatic tissue, although the prostate itself is nontender. Urodynamic studies may demonstrate incomplete relaxation of the bladder neck and prostatic urethra with diminished flow rates.

DRE usually reveals a normal prostate, though patients may have tenderness of pelvic floor musculature on palpation. Examination of the EPS shows leukocytes and lipid-laden macrophages.

Treatment of nonbacterial prostatitis is controversial. Some patients do improve with several weeks of oral antibiotics. In addition to fluoroquinolones, doxycycline may be added empirically to treat fastidious organisms such as *Chlamydia* that are not detected in initial cultures. Pentosan polysulfate (Elmiron) has shown promise in improving symptoms in 40% of patients. Alpha blockers (doxazosin, terazosin, or tamsulosin) are efficacious in patients with obstructive voiding symptoms. Antidepressants such as amitriptyline are useful in patients with significant pelvic and perineal pain.

Interstitial Cystitis

■ Epidemiology

Interstitial cystitis (IC) is a chronic disorder characterized by urinary frequency, nocturia, and suprapubic pain on bladder filling. Hematuria has been reported in 20% to 30% of cases. The disease occurs primarily in women aged 30 to 70 years. There is a 10:1 female to male preponderance.

■ Diagnosis

The diagnosis of IC is one of exclusion based on clinical and cystoscopic criteria. Patient have a chronic history of irritative bladder symptoms and pain. Urinary frequency occurs with small voided volumes. Physical examination fails to reveal any pertinent findings. Urinalysis and urine culture are often negative. Cystoscopy when performed reveals diffuse pinpoint submucosal hemorrhage after repeated bladder distension. If bladder biopsy is performed, inflammatory cells are often present, but no evidence of carcinoma in situ or transitional cell carcinoma is seen. Urodynamic studies often reveal sensory urgency with incomplete relaxation of the external urinary sphincter in voiding. Because IC is a diagnosis of exclusion, patients need to be worked up with a urinalysis, urine culture, voiding record, intravenous pyelogram, and cystoscopy.

■ Treatment

Treatment of IC often involves several different therapeutic options. Cystoscopy with hydrodistention under anesthesia has been effective in approximately 30% of patients. Intravesical installation of dimethyl sulfoxide (DMSO) is a useful treatment and gives temporary relief in approximately 50% of patients. Amitriptyline, a tricyclic antidepressant, is useful in the management of neuropathic pain. Its use in IC patients has been well described. Pentosan polysulfate (Elmiron) is a synthetic sulfated polysaccharide that is used to repair the glycosaminoglycan layer, which is thought to be deficient in IC. This agent improves pain and voiding symptoms in approximately 50% to 65% of patients. Anticholinergic agents are useful in the management of associated detrusor overactivity. Sacral nerve stimulation is reserved for patients who have failed medical therapy.

Epididymitis and Orchitis

Epididymitis is an inflammation of the epididymis. Most cases are due to ascending infection from the lower urinary tract. Increased pressure in the prostatic urethra during voiding allows infected urine to enter the ejaculatory ducts and traverse via the vas deferens to reach the epididymis. In men younger than 40 years, sexually transmitted pathogens such as *Neisseria gonorrhoeae* and *Chlamydia trachomatis* are common causes of epididymitis. In older men, *E. coli* is the most common organism.

Orchitis is an acute infection of the testis. Because the testis possesses a relatively high infection resistance, orchitis is rare without an initial epididymitis. The two major distinguishing etiologies of orchitis are blood-borne bacterial infection and viral infection. Pyogenic bacterial orchitis is usually secondary to bacterial involvement of the epididymis. The most common bacterial pathogens are *E. coli*, *Klebsiella pneumoniae*, and *Pseudomonas aeruginosa*. Viral orchitis is most commonly caused by mumps. This is rarely seen in prepubertal boys, but occurs in 20% to 30% of postpubertal boys with mumps.

■ Diagnosis

The clinical presentation of epididymitis and orchitis involves scrotal swelling and pain that is usually severe and develops rapidly. Symptoms and signs of cystitis, prostatitis, or urethritis may also be present. Physical examination reveals scrotal erythema and swelling. It is important to rule out testicular torsion, a urologic emergency, in a patient presenting with acute scrotal pain. Prehn's sign, alleviation of pain with scrotal elevation, is present in acute epididymitis but generally not in testicular torsion. It may be important to rule out testicular torsion by performing a duplex Doppler ultrasound study of the testicle. In cases of epididymitis, normal blood flow to the testicle is identified, and the involved epididymis is enlarged with hyperemia (increased blood flow).

In testicular torsion, no appreciable blood flow is identified in the involved testicle.

■ **Treatment**

Epididymo-orchitis related to *N. gonorrhoeae* or *C. trachomatis* should be treated with single-dose ceftriaxone or with a 10-day course of tetracycline or erythromycin. If an enteric pathogen is suspected, a 2-week course of broad-spectrum oral antibiotics such as trimethoprim-sulfamethoxazole is recommended. Additional supportive management includes bed rest, scrotal elevation, and pain medications.

Fournier's Gangrene

Fournier's gangrene is a rare, progressive, necrotizing fascitis of the genitalia or the perineum. It is a true urologic emergency and demands early recognition and prompt medical and surgical treatment.

■ **Risk Factors**

Increased risk for developing Fournier's gangrene is associated with conditions of immunodeficiency such as diabetes, malnutrition, alcoholism, intravenous drug abuse, hemodialysis, and use of steroid medications. Local trauma, including procedures and operations such as circumcision, penile prosthesis insertion, and vasectomy, may also increase risk.

■ **Pathogenesis**

The source of infection is either the genitourinary or gastrointestinal tract. Fournier's gangrene is a polymicrobial infection, with causative organisms including *E. coli*, *Bacteroides*, *Clostridium*, streptococci, and staphylococci. Ultimately, an obliterative endarteritis develops, and the ensuing cutaneous and subcutaneous vascular necrosis leads to localized ischemia and further bacterial proliferation. Rates of fascial destruction as high as 2 to 3 cm/h have been described. As gangrene develops, pain actually may subside as nerve tissue becomes necrotic.

■ **Diagnosis**

Patients present with irritation, itching, and erythema of the perineal region. The genital, perianal, or rectal discomfort is usually out of proportion to the physical examination findings. The skin overlying the affected region may be erythematous, edematous, cyanotic, bronzed, indurated, blistered, or even gangrenous.

A feculent odor may be present secondary to infection with anaerobic bacteria. Crepitus may be present, but its absence does not exclude the presence of *Clostridium* species or other gas-producing organisms.

■ Treatment

Initiation of prompt broad-spectrum intravenous antibiotic therapy is important because wound and tissue cultures often grow multiple aerobic and anaerobic organisms. Triple-antibiotic therapy that includes an aminoglycoside, penicillin derivative, and anaerobic coverage is recommended. Typically, ampicillin, gentamicin, and metronidazole are given intravenously. Prompt surgical wound débridement minimizes progression of necrosis. Multiple débridements in the operating room may be required to remove all necrotic tissue effectively. In some cases, diverting colostomy and suprapubic cystotomy are required to divert the fecal and urinary streams, respectively.

Sexually Transmitted Diseases

Urethritis and Cervicitis

Urethritis (inflammation of the urethra) is often caused by infection. It is characterized by purulent urethral discharge and dysuria. Cervicitis (inflammation of the cervix or endocervix) is characterized by a mucopurulent exudate visible in the endocervical canal or on an endocervical swab sample. Patients may present with vaginal discharge, but are often asymptomatic. Infectious causes of urethritis and cervicitis typically are sexually transmitted and categorized as gonococcal, due to *Neisseria gonorrhoeae*, or nongonococcal, due to *Chlamydia trachomatis*, *Ureaplasma urealyticum*, *Mycoplasma hominis*, or *Trichomonas vaginalis*. Urethritis usually resolves without complication, even if untreated, although it can result in urethral stricture or stenosis.

Gonococcal Urethritis

Gonococcal urethritis is the most frequently reported infectious disease in the United States. The offending organism is *N. gonorrhoeae*. Coinfection with *C. trachomatis* occurs in 20% of males infected with gonorrhea. Male patients usually present with purulent and copious urethral discharge associated with dysuria and urethral itching. Complications include epididymitis, prostatitis, and urethral strictures. Disseminated gonococcal infections present with macular skin lesions and multiarticular tenosynovitis.

■ Diagnosis

Diagnosis is usually made by visualizing intracellular gram-negative diplococci on Gram stain. *N. gonorrhea* should be cultured on Thayer-Martin media, although DNA amplification probes yield more rapid results and provide better sensitivity and specificity.

■ Treatment

Table 7-1 shows the current recommended treatment for gonococcal urethritis.

■ TABLE 7-1 Treatment Protocol for Urethritis, Cervicitis, and Nongonococcal Urethritis

Infection	Treatment
Gonococcal infections— uncomplicated urethral, cervical, or rectal infections	Ceftriaxone 125 mg IM single dose
	Ciprofloxacin 500 mg single dose
	Levofloxacin 250 mg single dose + azithromycin 1 g single dose
	Doxycycline 100 mg BID for 7 days
Nongonococcal urethritis	Azithromycin 1 g single dose
	Doxycycline 100 mg BID for 7 days
Recurrent or persistent urethritis	Metronidazole 2 g single dose + erythromycin base 500 mg QID for 7 days
	Consider treatment for interstitial cystitis/ chronic prostatitis as necessary

Nongonococcal Urethritis

The most common cause of nongonococcal urethritis (NGU) is *C. trachomatis*, an obligate intracellular organism with a tendency to infect only squamocolumnar and columnar epithelia. Urethral discharge is less purulent than that seen in gonococcal urethritis, usually thin and clear, although often it is not associated with any discharge. Complications in women include pelvic inflammatory disease (PID), tubal scarring, ectopic pregnancy, and infertility. Reiter's syndrome is a noninfectious complication of NGU and is defined as a triad of arthritis, conjunctivitis, and urethritis.

■ Diagnosis

A presumptive diagnosis of NGU is made with more than 4 polymorphonuclear (PMN) cells per oil immersion field and a negative Gram stain. DNA amplification probes can aid in diagnosis.

■ Treatment

Table 7-1 shows the current recommended treatment.

Trichomoniasis

Trichomonas vaginalis is a flagellated protozoan and the most common parasite leading to urethritis. Infection in males is usually asymptomatic. In female patients, there is a characteristic greenish, malodorous vaginal discharge. Patients usually present with soreness, itching, and dysuria.

■ Diagnosis

A sample of the discharge treated with 10% potassium hydroxide (KOH) yields a fishy odor and has a pH greater than 4.5. Microscopic examination will demonstrate highly motile flagellated trichomonads and leukocytes.

■ Treatment

Metronidazole as a 2-g single dose is associated with a 95% cure rate. Some increased resistance to metronidazole has been observed. This product must be avoided during the first 20 weeks of pregnancy. In these cases, clotrimazole vaginal suppositories should be used. Sexual partners should be treated empirically to prevent recurrence.

Syphilis

Syphilis is caused by the spirochete *Treponema pallidum*, and is characterized by three clinical stages: primary, secondary, and tertiary. Sexual transmission occurs only when mucocutaneous lesions are present.

Primary syphilis is characterized by a painless chancre with an indurated edge that often remains unnoticed by the patient. The incubation period is approximately 3 weeks. Secondary syphilis appears 4 to 8 weeks after the resolution of the primary lesion and is characterized by constitutional symptoms including fever and malaise, distinctive truncal and palmar erythematous rash, and condylomata latum, a highly infectious weeping, verrucous sore. The second stage resolves if untreated, and the disease may enter a latency period of 2 to 40 years. Approximately 25% of patients develop tertiary syphilis, which may affect the cardiovascular (CV) and central nervous systems. CV findings include aortic insufficiency and aortic aneurysm. Neurosyphilis is characterized by tabes dorsalis, Argyll-Robertson pupils, and dementia. Patients with tertiary syphilis may present with a sensory neurogenic bladder.

■ Diagnosis

Early syphilis is diagnosed by darkfield microscopy and direct fluorescent antibody tests of the scrapings from the base of the ulcer. In addition, presumptive diagnosis can be made through two serologic tests: nontreponemal, such as the Venereal Disease Research Laboratory (VDRL) and rapid plasma reagent (RPR) tests, or treponemal, such as the fluorescent treponemal antibody absorption (FTA-ABS) test and microagglutination assay for antibody to

■ TABLE 7-2 Recommended Treatment Regimen for Syphilis

Stage or Type	Treatment
Primary and secondary	Benzathine penicillin G 2.4 million units IM as a single dose
Tertiary (except neurosyphilis)	Benzathine penicillin G 2.4 million units IM weekly for 3 weeks
Neurosyphilis	Procaine penicillin 2.4 million units IM daily for 10–14 days + Probenecid 500 mg PO QID for 10–14 days
Latent syphilis	Early: Benzathine penicillin G 2.4 million units IM as a single dose Late: Benzathine penicillin G 2.4 million units IM weekly for 3 weeks

T. pallidum (MHA-TP). VDRL and RPR serve as good screening tests, although false positives may occur in patients with systemic lupus erythematosus, arthritis, and narcotic addiction. Diagnosis is confirmed with the more sensitive MHA-TP or FTA-ABS. Nontreponemal antibody titers are reported quantitatively and usually correlate with disease activity, whereas most patients with reactive treponemal tests remain reactive for life.

■ Treatment

Treatment options for various stages are outlined in Table 7-2. A follow-up visit 6 months after treatment should show a fourfold decline in antibody titers. If such a decline in titer levels is not noted, evaluation for neurosyphilis should be undertaken. Neurosyphilis requires a more aggressive therapy than primary and secondary syphilis. Desensitization is recommended for patients allergic to penicillin.

Chancroid

Chancroid is an acute ulcerative disease with inguinal adenopathy. It is caused by *Haemophilus ducreyi*, a gram-negative facultative bacillus. Although it was infrequently diagnosed in the past, it is now endemic in many parts of the United States. The organism is transmitted by direct contact through the skin, presumably through minor abrasions. After an incubation period of 2 to 10 days, a papule or pustule erupts that erodes to form a painful ulcer with ragged margins. The ulcer may be quite deep, and more than one-half of patients have multiple ulcers.

■ Diagnosis

Most patients present with the complaint of one or more painful genital ulcers, associated with tender, enlarged lymph nodes in the groin. The lymphadenitis usually appears about 1 to 2 weeks after the primary lesion. The combination of a painful genital ulcer with suppurative inguinal adenopathy is pathognomonic. Definitive diagnosis requires identification of *H. ducreyi* on a specialized culture media. The classic description of *H. ducreyi* on Gram stain is that of a "school of fish" with small, pleomorphic gram-negative rods, although the sensitivity of Gram staining is less than 80%. Because there are few diagnostic tests available for infection with *H. ducreyi*, diagnosis is made via exclusion of syphilis and herpes simplex virus.

■ Treatment

The recommended antimicrobial treatment is as follows: azithromycin 1 g as a single oral dose, or ceftriaxone 250 mg as a single intramuscular dose, or ciprofloxacin 500 mg twice a day for 3 days. Follow-up is recommended after 3 to 7 days to assess improvement. Occasionally, patients require incision and drainage of fluctuant inguinal nodes. Patients should be tested for syphilis and retested 3 months later if the initial test result is negative. The reason for this testing is that approximately 10% of patients with chancroid are coinfected with either *T. pallidum* or herpes simplex virus.

Lymphogranuloma Venereum

Lymphogranuloma venereum (LGV) is caused by *C. trachomatis* serotypes L1, L2, and L3. LGV occurs rarely in the United States. The organism gains entrance to the body through skin breaks and abrasions, or it crosses the epithelial cells of mucous membranes. The organism travels via the lymphatics to multiply within mononuclear phagocytes in regional lymph nodes.

■ Diagnosis

The primary lesion of LGV occurs after an incubation period of 3 to 21 days following an exposure. The initial lesion may be a painless papule, shallow erosion, or ulcer. Tender inguinal or femoral lymphadenopathy, often unilateral, is the most common clinical manifestation in heterosexual men. Homosexual men and women may present with perirectal and pelvic lymph node involvement. Diagnosis is made by serologic testing.

■ Treatment

The goal of therapy is to cure the microbiological disease and prevent tissue destruction. Doxycycline 100 mg twice a day for 21 days is the preferred treatment. Tissue retraction and scarring is still possible even after effective antibiotic treatment. Inguinal adenopathy may require needle aspiration and drainage to prevent inguinal or femoral ulcerations. Patients must be followed until their clinical symptoms resolve.

Granuloma Inguinale

Granuloma inguinale is caused by *Calymmatobacterium granulomatis*, a pleomorphic gram-negative bacillus. The incubation period may range from 1 week to 3 months. This infection is rare in the United States, but is endemic in Western New Guinea, the Caribbean, Southern India, South Africa, and Southeast Asia. Clinically, granuloma inguinale presents as a painless ulcer with a clean, friable base and distinct raised margins. The ulcers typically appear beefy red and are extremely friable.

■ Diagnosis

The causative organism is extremely difficult to culture. The most effective method of diagnosis is direct visualization of the organism within macrophages as intracytoplasmic inclusions, known as **Donovan bodies,** on tissue crush preparations. Molecular diagnostic tests are currently in development.

■ Treatment

The recommended antibiotics are either trimethoprim-sulfamethoxazole or doxycycline. Alternatives include ciprofloxacin, erythromycin, or azithromycin. The antibiotic should be given for at least 3 weeks and then continued until clearing is evident. Patients should be reevaluated after a few days of treatment to check their response. If lesions have not responded adequately, an aminoglycoside may be added. Treatment should be continued until all lesions have healed. Relapse can occur as late as 18 months after initial therapy.

Condyloma Acuminata (Venereal Warts)

Genital warts are caused by human papillomavirus (HPV) infection. Although more than 70 types of HPV have been isolated, 90% of genital warts are caused by HPV types 6 and 11, which are the least likely to have cancer-causing potential. Other less common types have been strongly associated with premalignant lesions such as cervical dysplasia and malignant lesions such as squamous cell carcinoma of the cervix, erythroplasia of Queyrat, and Bowen's disease of the penis. HPV-16 alone is responsible for about 50% of cervical cancers, and types 16, 18, 31, 33, and 45 together account for 80% of cervical cancers.

■ Diagnosis

Genital warts are flesh-colored or gray growths found in the genital area and anal region in both men and women. Condyloma acuminata is the most common sexually transmitted disease caused by a virus. Infection with genital warts may not be obvious. Men and women with genital warts will often complain of painless bumps, itching, and discharge.

In men, genital warts can infect the urethra, penis, scrotum, and rectal area. The warts can appear as soft, raised cauliflower-like masses with a surface that can be smooth or rough with many fingerlike projections. It is necessary to carefully examine the external genitalia, since some lesions are hidden by hair or are in the inner aspect of the uncircumcised foreskin. In women, genital warts have a similar appearance and usually occur in the moist areas of the labia minora and vaginal opening. It is necessary to examine the vaginal canal, cervix, and anorectal area for asymptomatic lesions.

Diagnosis is often based on findings from the history and physical examination. Infected areas usually turn white following application of 5% acetic acid solution for 10 minutes. Rarely, a biopsy might be necessary to confirm the diagnosis. A routine Pap smear should always be done to look for evidence of HPV infection and abnormal cells on the cervix.

■ Treatment

No single treatment is effective in eliminating warts or preventing their recurrence. Genital warts may spontaneously disappear in about 10% to 20% of people over a period of 3 to 4 months, although recurrence is frequently inevitable. Patient-applied treatments include a 0.5% solution of podofilox gel applied to the lesions twice a day for 3 days, followed by 4 days off therapy. This process can be repeated for up to four cycles. Imiquimod 5% cream can also be applied to the lesions at bedtime 3 times per week for up to 16 weeks.

Surgical removal can be done as an office procedure with local anesthesia. Surgery is usually performed when the warts are small in size and number. Of all the treatment techniques, surgery has the highest success rate and lowest recurrence rate. Cryotherapy is a technique that treats the wart using liquid nitrogen, but is often very painful. Several medications exist for treating genital warts and can be used as an alternative to surgical removal.

Genital Herpes Simplex

Genital herpes simplex (HSV) affects approximately 55 million people in the United States. It is caused by two serotypes: HSV-1 and HSV-2. Multiple painful vesicles with an erythematous base are characteristic of early HSV infections. Patients present with local symptoms of burning, pain, pruritus, and lymphadenopathy and constitutional symptoms of malaise and flu-like symptoms. Recurrences of herpetic lesions are less severe, with fewer constitutional symptoms. Women tend to have more severe symptoms, but symptoms in men are of longer duration. Risk factors for recurrence include stress, fatigue, immunosuppression, pregnancy, and menstruation.

■ Diagnosis

Diagnosis can be made via a Tzanck smear of the lesion, demonstrating multinucleated giant cells with a basophilic nuclear rim and paler-staining central nucleus. In addition, enzyme-linked immunosorbent assay (ELISA) and direct immunofluorescence provide a definitive diagnosis.

■ Treatment

Genital herpes is an incurable and recurrent viral infection. Oral antiviral agents may ease local and constitutional symptoms and reduce the number of recurrences. Three antiviral drugs have proved of benefit in randomized clinical trials: acyclovir, valacyclovir, and famciclovir. Topical treatment with acyclovir is less effective than systemic treatments. Table 7-3 lists treatment options for genital herpes.

A summary of the differential diagnosis of sexually transmitted diseases and genital ulcers is provided in Table 7-4.

■ TABLE 7-3 Treatment of Genital Herpes

Occurrence	Treatment
First episode	Acyclovir 400 mg PO TID for 7–10 days Acyclovir 200 mg PO 5 times a day for 7–10 days Famciclovir 250 mg PO TID for 7–10 days Valacyclovir 1 g PO BID for 7–10 days
Recurrent episodes	Acyclovir 400 mg PO TID for 5 days Acyclovir 200 mg PO 5 times a day for 5 days Famciclovir 125 mg PO BID for 5 days Valacyclovir 500 mg PO BID for 5 days
Daily suppression therapy	Acyclovir 400 mg PO BID Famciclovir 250 mg PO BID Valacyclovir 250 mg PO BID

■ TABLE 7-4 Differential Diagnosis of Sexually Transmitted Diseases and Genital Ulcers: A Review

Disease	Etiology	Incubation Time	Lesion	Diagnostic Tests
Syphilitic chancre	*Treponema pallidum*	2–4 wk	Painful ulcer	Darkfield microscopy, VDRL, RPR, FTA-ABS
Chancroid	*Haemophilus ducreyi*	3–10 days	Very painful ulcer	Selective medium culture for *H. ducreyi*, and Gram stain
Granuloma inguinale	*Calymmatobacterium granulomata*	2–3 mo	Minimally painful superficial ulcer	None
Lympho-granuloma	*Chlamydia trachomatis*	3–21 days	None	None
Herpes	Herpes virus type 2	Unknown	Multiple superficial vesicles, with local burning or itching	Isolation of virus

VDRL, Venereal Disease Research Laboratory; RPR, rapid plasma reagent; FTA-ABS, fluorescent treponemal antibody absorption.

8 Genitourinary Oncology

RENAL PARENCHYMAL NEOPLASMS

Benign Tumors

■ Renal Adenomas

Renal adenomas are usually small, well-differentiated benign tumors of the renal cortex. They are usually asymptomatic and are often seen in the kidney at autopsy or incidentally during workup for an unrelated disease. A small proportion may undergo malignant change to renal cell carcinoma (RCC) and therefore should be treated as RCC, especially if they are larger than 3 cm. Nephron-sparing surgery is usually adequate for removing these tumors.

■ Renal Oncocytoma

Renal oncocytomas are relatively benign tumors derived from proximal tubular cells. They constitute about 3% to 5% of all renal tumors and account for approximately 500 cases per year. The male-to-female ratio is 2:1. Grossly, they have a well-defined fibrous capsule and are brown or tan. Histologically, they are composed predominantly of well-differentiated granular eosinophilic cells arranged in a tubular, alveolar, or papillary pattern. Oncocytomas are usually discovered incidentally, but also may present with hematuria or flank pain.

Oncocytomas cannot be differentiated from RCC radiographically. On computed tomographic (CT) scan, there may be a variable appearance of a central scar, especially in large tumors. Angiographically, there is often a "spoke-wheel" appearance to the vessels.

The definitive diagnosis is made by histologic examination of the tumor. Because a preoperative definitive diagnosis is difficult to make and because high-grade oncocytomas may be found with elements of renal cell carcinoma, radical or partial nephrectomy is the treatment of choice.

■ Angiomyolipoma (Renal Hamartoma)

Angiomyolipoma (AML) is a benign renal neoplasm composed of fat, blood vessels, and smooth muscle and is often seen in patients with tuberous sclerosis (TS). The majority (>75%) of cases of AML present sporadically and commonly occur in middle-aged women. Twenty percent of AML cases are associated with TS, and more than 50% of patients with TS have AML. TS is an autosomal dominant syndrome characterized by mental retardation, adenoma sebaceum, and seizure disorder. Renal lesions tend to be small, multiple, and often bilateral when associated with TS. Conversely, non-TS lesions are larger and unilateral.

Most AML lesions are asymptomatic and present as incidental findings on ultrasound (US) or CT scan. When symptomatic, AML can present with hematuria or flank pain or both and can be associated with a palpable abdominal mass. Preoperative diagnosis is often possible with imaging studies. On US, a characteristic bright echo pattern is seen due to the high fat content of these tumors. Similarly, CT scans show the fatty tumor as a low-density mass, which is often diagnostic.

Asymptomatic lesions that are smaller than 4 cm can usually be observed. The major concern in lesions larger than 4 cm is the risk of hemorrhage. Therefore, if a tumor is larger than 4 cm or is symptomatic (i.e., pain, bleeding), treatment may include partial or total nephrectomy or selective embolization.

Renal Cell Carcinoma

■ Epidemiology

Renal cell carcinoma is the most common renal malignancy, and accounts for about 3% of all adult neoplasms and approximately 85% of all primary malignant renal tumors. Males are affected twice as commonly as females. The incidence may also vary with race, since black men demonstrate a higher incidence that those of other races. RCC most commonly occurs in the fifth to seventh decade, with a mean age of 58. Patients with a history of von Hippel-Lindau (VHL) syndrome generally present at a younger age (<50 years).

■ Risk Factors

Various risk factors have been implicated in the development of RCC. Acquired risk factors include history of tobacco use, asbestos and heavy metal exposure, abuse of the analgesic phenacetin, renal transplantation, and renal cystic disease from dialysis. Hereditary risk factors include polycystic kidney disease, VHL syndrome, and tuberous sclerosis. VHL syndrome is an autosomal dominant condition characterized by cerebellar hemangioblastomas, pheochromocytoma, pancreatic and renal cysts, retinal angiomas, and a predisposition to a variety of neoplasms, including RCC.

In fact, RCC develops in nearly 40% of patients with VHL syndrome and is a major cause of death among these patients.

Hereditary papillary renal cell carcinoma (HPRCC) was recently described and is characterized by multiple bilateral renal tumors that have a papillary histologic appearance. In contrast to VHL, HPRCC has no neoplastic manifestations outside of the kidneys.

Acquired cystic disease of the kidneys is a well-described condition associated with multiple bilateral renal cysts in patients with end-stage renal disease. Such patients have a 30-fold increase in development of RCC if they have cystic changes in their kidneys. Up to 10% of people with acquired cystic disease of the kidneys develop RCC.

■ Pathology

Grossly, these tumors comprise a discrete mass within the cortex of the kidney and have a homogeneous yellowish appearance on cut section. On microscopy, several histologic subtypes have been described: **clear cell** (75%), **chromophilic** (15%), and **chromophobic** (5%). Most clear cell carcinoma originates in the proximal renal tubular epithelium and is characterized by round or polygonal cells with abundant cytoplasm containing glycogen. Clear cell carcinoma results from a deletion of chromosome 3p. Chromophilic, or papillary, RCC tends to be bilateral and is more commonly found in patients with end-stage renal failure and acquired renal cystic disease. It is also associated with trisomy 7 and 17 and loss of Y chromosome. Chromophobic carcinoma is characterized by large polygonal cells with a pale reticular cytoplasm. Papillary and chromophobic RCC tend to originate from more distal parts of the nephron. In addition, VHL mutations and chromosome 3 abnormalities are uncommon with these tumors. A sarcomatoid variant can occur in all histologic cell types of RCC and tends to have a poorer prognosis.

■ Clinical Manifestations

Signs and Symptoms

Only 11% of patients present with the classic triad of hematuria, flank pain, and a palpable mass. The finding of a palpable mass is usually indicative of advanced disease. Forty percent of the cases are found incidentally on imaging studies typically ordered for some other abdominal symptoms. Tumor extension into the left renal vein may result in an acute onset of a varicocele, and involvement of the inferior vena cava (IVC) may produce bilateral leg edema. Symptoms secondary to metastases include bone pain (from lung, brain, and bone metastases), dyspnea, cough, seizure, or headaches.

■ TABLE 8-1 Paraneoplastic Syndromes Associated with Renal Cell Carcinoma

Syndrome	Cause
Anemia	Hematuria, chronic disease
Polycythemia	Ectopic secretion of erythropoietin
Hypertension	Ectopic secretion of renin
Hypoglycemia	Ectopic secretion of insulin
Cushing's syndrome	Ectopic secretion of ACTH
Hypercalcemia	Ectopic secretion of parathyroid hormone-like substance
Gynecomastia, amenorrhea, baldness	Ectopic secretion of gonadotropins
Hepatic dysfunction (Stauffer's syndrome)	Unknown
Pyrexia, night sweats	Unknown

ACTH, adrenocorticotropic hormone.

Paraneoplastic syndromes have been associated with RCC. Table 8-1 lists some of the common syndromes associated with RCC. Systemic symptoms include hypercalcemia in 20% (ectopic parathyroid hormone production), reversible elevation of liver function test results (LFTs) in 3% to 20% (Stauffer's syndrome), erythrocytosis in 3% to 10% (erythropoietin secretion), and hypertension in up to 40% (renin secretion). Overall, these manifestations can occur in 10% to 40% of patients with RCC.

Physical examination may reveal a mass in the flank region, but is usually nonspecific. A complete exam is necessary to check for signs of metastatic disease, such as supraclavicular adenopathy. Lung is the most common site of metastases, followed by liver, bone, ipsilateral lymph nodes, and adrenal glands.

■ Diagnostic Evaluation

Laboratory Studies
Urinalysis is positive for hematuria in 60% of the patients. Urine culture and cytology are usually normal. A complete blood count (CBC) and serum chemistries may reveal signs of paraneoplastic syndromes such as hypercalcemia, elevation of LFTs, or erythrocytosis. The erythrocyte sedimentation rate (ESR) is elevated in up to 75% of the patients. Anemia occurs in 30% of RCC patients. This is usually not related to blood loss and is normocytic in nature.

Imaging Studies
CT scan is the most sensitive and cost-effective single imaging study in diagnosing RCC. Findings include a heterogenous

low-density mass in the cortex of the kidney that enhances with intravenous contrast. In addition, CT scan of the chest and abdomen can help in the clinical staging of the disease, such as nodal enlargement or metastases.

Intravenous pyelography (IVP) can also be used in the evaluation of hematuria and is 75% accurate in the diagnosis of RCC. Calcification overlying the renal shadow, renal displacement, and poor visualization of the kidney increase the probability of cancer. Questionable findings on IVP can be confirmed with a CT scan.

Ultrasonography is useful in the diagnosis of renal cysts. It may also be useful in the diagnosis of renal mass lesions. US may also be able to detect invasion of tumor thrombus into the IVC. Fine-needle aspiration (FNA) has a limited role in diagnosing RCC. FNA is rarely performed and is only helpful in differentiating primary RCC from metastatic tumors to the kidney.

■ Treatment

If the renal mass is confined to the kidney without any evidence of metastases, radical nephrectomy is the treatment of choice. This procedure involves the complete removal of the Gerota's fascia and resection of the kidney, together with the upper ureter and perirenal fat, with or without the ipsilateral adrenal gland and para-aortic lymph nodes. The goal is to achieve removal of the kidney and take a wide margin of normal tissue. The likelihood of local recurrence after radical nephrectomy is approximately 3%. Between 20% and 30% of patients undergoing radical nephrectomy with lymph node dissection are found to have pathologic evidence of metastatic disease. Some advocate the use of angioinfarction prior to nephrectomy in cases of very large tumors in an attempt to decrease blood loss during the subsequent nephrectomy.

Currently, trials of laparoscopic nephrectomy are underway. This technique is being used for patients with localized tumors. Recent data suggest this procedure has a quicker recovery time, less operative blood loss, and equivalent efficacy compared with radical nephrectomy.

If the tumor is small (<4 cm), bilateral, or if the patient has a single functioning kidney, partial nephrectomy (nephron-sparing surgery) is the best option. Local recurrence of tumor in the same kidney ranges from 0% to 10%. Long-term follow-up indicates an outcome similar to radical nephrectomy.

New therapeutic treatments currently under study for small, incidentally discovered renal masses include cryoablation, high-intensity focused ultrasound (HIFU), and radiofrequency ablation. These techniques may be applicable in patients with multiple small lesions or in older patients who have multiple medical problems.

Metastatic RCC has a very poor prognosis, with an average survival of 4 months after the diagnosis is made. RCC is refractory to nearly all chemotherapeutic agents, and radiation therapy has not proved to be of any benefit in treating metastatic RCC. Surgery is reserved for intractable symptoms such as bleeding and pain. However, there is some belief that radical nephrectomy even in the face of metastatic disease may improve response rates with subsequent chemotherapy or treatment with biologic response modifiers (interferon-alpha). In patients with synchronous metastasis (kidney and ipsilateral lung), nephrectomy and resection of the metastatic focus may improve survival. Trials of hormonal agents (antiestrogenic agents) for RCC have been poor, with response rates ranging from 0% to 30%. RCC is one of the most chemoresistant tumors, which may be related to the presence of the P-glycoprotein. The response rate with this form of therapy is approximately 5%.

The use of biologic response modifiers in the treatment of RCC shows some promise. Studies using interferon-alpha and interleukin suggest a 15% to 30% response rate. However, these therapies are associated with various toxicities that may limit their use.

Table 8-2 presents the TNM classification system for RCC. Table 8-3 presents the staging system for RCC and approximate prognosis.

Tumors of the Renal Pelvis and Ureter

■ Epidemiology

Tumors of the renal pelvis are uncommon and account for approximately 8% of all renal tumors and less than 5% of all urothelial tumors. Ureteral tumors are even more uncommon, occurring with one-fourth the incidence of renal pelvis tumors. Similar to bladder cancer, the male-to-female ratio of incidence is 3:1. The mean age of occurrence is 65 years. Patients with multiple, recurrent superficial bladder cancers are at risk for the development of ureteral and renal pelvic tumors. The cumulative risk of such cancers is approximately 10% at 5 years of follow-up.

■ Risk Factors

Many of the risk factors for developing transitional cell carcinoma (TCC) of the renal pelvis and ureter are similar to those of bladder TCC, including smoking and occupational hazards (see the risk factors section for bladder tumors, later in this chapter).

■ TABLE 8-2 TNM Staging System for Renal Cell Carcinoma

T: Primary Tumor

TX	Primary tumor cannot be assessed
T0	No evidence of a primary tumor
T1	Tumor <7 cm and confined to the kidney
T2	Tumor >7 cm and confined to the kidney
T3	Tumor extends into major veins or invades adrenal gland or perinephric tissues but not beyond Gerota's fascia
T3a	Tumor invades adrenal gland or perinephric tissues but not beyond Gerota's fascia
T3b	Tumor grossly extends into renal vein or vena cava
T3c	Tumor grossly extends into renal vein above the diaphragm
T4	Tumor invades beyond Gerota's fascia

N: Regional Lymph Nodes

NX	Regional nodes cannot be assessed
N0	No regional lymph node metastases
N1	Metastases in a single regional lymph node 2 cm or less
N2	Metastases in more than a single regional lymph node

M: Distant Metastases

MX	Distant metastases cannot be assessed
M1	No distant metastases
M2	Distant metastases

Upper tract TCC does not have a genetic or hereditary pattern, but there is an association between upper tract TCC and Balkan nephropathy. This latter condition is a degenerative nephropathy confined to rural areas of Balkan countries and is associated with

■ TABLE 8-3 Staging of Renal Cell Carcinoma and Prognosis

Stage	Findings	5-Year Survival (%)
I	Tumor confined to kidney parenchyma No involvement of perinephric fat, renal vein, or regional lymph nodes	91–100
II	Tumor involves perinephric fat but confined to Gerota's fascia	74–96
IIIa	Tumor involves main renal vein or inferior vena cava	59–70
IIIb	Tumor involves regional lymph nodes	
IIIc	Tumor involves both vessels and regional lymph nodes	
IVa	Tumor involves adjacent organs other than the adrenal glands (colon, pancreas, etc.)	16–32
IVb	Distant metastases	

an increased incidence of TCC. The exact mechanism of tumor formation in this condition is poorly understood.

■ Pathology

The renal pelvis and ureter are lined by transitional epithelium. Therefore, TCC is the most common tumor, accounting for greater than 90% of upper tract urothelial tumors. Squamous cell carcinoma constitutes 1% to 7% of upper tract urothelial tumors. It is usually seen in patients with a long-standing history of chronic inflammation, such as those with infected staghorn calculi.

TCC has a high rate of recurrence and a very high seeding potential distally in the urinary tract. Approximately 30% to 75% of patients with upper tract urothelial tumors develop bladder tumors at some point in the future. Other common sites of metastases include regional lymph nodes, lung, and bone.

■ Clinical Manifestations

Signs and Symptoms

Gross or microscopic hematuria (75%) is the most common clinical presentation. Flank pain, if present, usually results from gradual distention of the collecting system secondary to obstruction by the tumor. Also, hydronephrosis may cause a palpable flank mass. Irritative voiding symptoms are present in approximately 10% of patients. Symptoms of metastatic disease include weight loss, anorexia, and lethargy. Some patients with metastatic disease present with supraclavicular or inguinal adenopathy.

■ Diagnostic Evaluation

The imaging study of choice is an intravenous pyelogram. Abnormalities seen on IVP include hydronephrosis, intraluminal filling defect, and nonvisualization of the collecting system. When IVP is inconclusive, a retrograde pyelogram (RPG) may assist in a more accurate visualization of the collecting system. An ultrasound, CT, or MRI study may not be sensitive enough to detect tumors of the renal pelvis. Direct visualization with ureteroscopy allows for inspection of the filling defects and for obtaining biopsies for cytologic evaluation.

Laboratory Studies and Cytopathology

Hematuria is identified in most patients. Some patients present with pyuria and bacteruria. Washed ureteral catheter cytologies can further aid in the diagnosis. Voided urine samples obtained for cytopathology lack sensitivity, especially for low-grade tumors, for which cytology is read as normal in as many as 80% of patients. Sensitivity increases for higher-grade tumors, which tend to shed more tumor cells. Cytology has an overall accuracy of 83% in diagnosing patients with grade IV disease but can miss significant numbers of low-grade cancers.

■ Treatment

The gold-standard treatment for nonmetastatic disease is a nephro-ureterectomy with excision of the bladder cuff. This involves removing the kidney and the ipsilateral ureter because of a high incidence of subsequent recurrence in the ureteric stump. Tumors of the distal ureter may be treated with distal ureterectomy and ureteral reimplantation into the bladder, provided that there is no proximal evidence of TCC.

In metastatic disease, treatment is combination chemotherapy using methotrexate, vinblastine, doxorubicin (Adriamycin), and cisplatin. Palliative surgery or renal artery embolization may be necessary for recurring hematuria. TCC of the upper tract is relatively resistant to radiation therapy.

Bladder Tumors

Bladder cancer is the second most common malignancy of the genitourinary tract. It is the fourth most common cancer in men and the eighth most common in women. It tends to metastasize to liver, lung, bone, adrenal glands, and bowel.

■ Epidemiology

The median age at diagnosis is 68 years, and the incidence increases with age. It is rare before the age of 40. Bladder cancer is twice as common in whites as in blacks. The male-to-female ratio is 3:1, although the number of cases has been increasing in women, possibly due to increased occupational exposure or smoking.

■ Risk Factors

Increasing age is a risk factor since the peak incidence of bladder tumors occurs in the seventh decade. Cigarette smoking carries a fourfold increased risk and accounts for a majority of the cases. Certain occupational exposure to chemicals has also been implicated in the development of bladder tumors. This includes exposure to aniline dyes and aromatic amines in the petroleum, dye, chemical, rubber, leather, and printing industries. Treatment with cyclophosphamide and pelvic radiation therapy for other neoplasms also carries a high risk of developing muscle-invasive tumors. Minimal data exist linking the use of artificial sweeteners, coffee, and tea to developing cancer. A previous history of

■ TABLE 8-4 TNM Staging for Bladder Cancer

Stage	Characteristics
CIS	Carcinoma in situ, high-grade dysplasia, confined to the epithelium
Ta	Papillary tumor confined to the epithelium
T1	Tumor invasion into the lamina propria
T2	Tumor invasion into the muscularis propria
T3	Tumor involvement of the perivesical fat
T4	Tumor involvement of adjacent organs such as prostate, rectum, or pelvic sidewall
N+	Lymph node metastasis
M+	Distant metastasis

renal pelvic or urothelial cancer increases risk by 20%. Risk factors for squamous cell carcinomas and adenocarcinomas of the bladder are discussed in the pathology section. The TNM staging system for bladder cancer is provided in Table 8-4.

■ Pathology

Transitional Cell Carcinoma
Transitional cell carcinoma accounts for more than 90% of bladder tumors in the United States. Staging is based on the depth of invasion of tumor into bladder epithelium and is necessary to determine the treatment options. The TNM staging system divides bladder tumors into carcinoma in situ (CIS), superficial carcinoma, and invasive carcinoma. Histologic grading is divided into three groups: well, moderately, and poorly differentiated. Grossly, they may appear sessile, papillary, infiltrating, nodular, or of mixed type. TCC commonly presents as a papillary, exophytic lesion with a thin fibrovascular stalk. The recurrence rate for superficial TCC is quite high, and as many as 80% of patients have at least one recurrence. On the other hand, muscle-invasive tumors tend to be nodular or sessile and are usually poorly differentiated or of high grade. Approximately 50% of all muscle-invasive bladder cancer may have occult metastases at the time of diagnosis. CIS is characterized by a velvety patch of erythematous mucosa and high-grade dysplasia of the bladder epithelium and is associated with a poorer prognosis.

Squamous Cell Carcinoma
Squamous cell carcinoma (SCC) accounts for between 5% and 10% of all bladder cancers in the United States. Incidence is increased in bladders with a history of chronic inflammation secondary to ova of *Schistosoma haematobium*, stones, and indwelling catheters. Schistosomiasis is more prevalent in the Middle East

and parts of Africa, including Egypt. Histologic characteristics of pure SCC are squamous "pearls," intercellular bridges, and keratinizing epithelium. A majority of SCCs are invasive at the time of diagnosis.

Adenocarcinomas

Adenocarcinoma of the bladder accounts for 2% of all bladder cancers. It usually arises from the urachus and remnants of the allantois in the dome of the bladder. Other risk factors include a history of congenital bladder exstrophy. On histologic studies, mucus-secreting glandular elements with a signet ring pattern are seen. Similar to squamous cell carcinomas, lesions are usually aggressive and high-grade compared with those of TCC. The 5-year survival rate is about 40%.

■ Clinical Manifestations

Signs and Symptoms

The most common presenting symptom of bladder cancer is either gross or microscopic hematuria. Irritative voiding symptoms such as increased frequency of urination, dysuria, and urgency may also indicate bladder cancer. Advanced disease may present with weight loss, inguinal adenopathy, and lower abdominal and bone pain. Physical examination is usually benign, although a large bladder tumor may be palpable in the suprapubic region. Bimanual examination may reveal bladder fixation to the pelvic side wall, rectum, or vagina.

■ Diagnostic Evaluation

Both the upper and lower urinary tract need to be evaluated. An upper tract study may include renal ultrasound, CT scan, or an intravenous pyelogram. A lower tract study (cystoscopy) is necessary for evaluation of the bladder and urethra.

Laboratory Studies

A urinalysis and urine culture are important as initial tests because a urinary tract infection may cause hematuria and is usually associated with irritative voiding symptoms. A complete blood count is necessary to exclude anemia secondary to chronic blood loss. In patients with a high risk of bladder cancer (age, smoking, occupational history), urine may be sent for cytologic examination. Urine cytology has a high sensitivity rate (>90%) for high-grade tumors, but only a sensitivity of 50% to 75% for grade I or II tumors. In addition, bladder tumor antigens released from the extracellular matrix of bladder tumors into voided urine may be detected using the bladder tumor antigen (BTA) test, which detects antigens to the urothelial basement membrane, or the nuclear matrix protein (NMP) 22 test, which detects antigens to nuclear proteins. Although the sensitivities of these newer tests are higher for lower-grade tumors compared with urine cytology, the specificities still remain low.

■ Treatment

Superficial Tumors

Superficial bladder cancer is initially treated by transurethral resection of bladder tumor (TURBT). Patients are then followed closely to determine recurrence. Multiple, large, or recurring tumors are potential candidates for intravesical chemotherapy. The most common agent used is bacille Calmette-Guérin (BCG), which is a live attenuated strain derived from *Mycobacterium bovis*. BCG causes local nonspecific immune response to the tumor proteins in the bladder by upregulating cytokines such as IL-6 and IL-8. It is usually administered weekly over a period of 6 weeks. Maintenance therapy can be given every 3 to 6 months. BCG therapy reduces recurrences by about 30% but has little, if any, effect on progression of the tumor. BCG typically causes mild systemic symptoms such as low-grade fever with myalgias that resolve within 24 to 48 hours. Rarely, it can cause an acute disseminated tuberculosis-like illness if it enters the bloodstream, manifesting as high persistent fever. In such cases multiagent antituberculosis therapy is started. BCG therapy is contraindicated in the presence of hematuria or following a traumatic catheterization.

Other intravesical agents currently used in BCG-refractory cases are thiotepa, mitomycin C, and doxorubicin. Thiotepa is an alkylating agent that is associated with a 55% complete response rate. Side effects that limit its use include mild cystitis after administration. More significant side effects include myelosuppression. Mitomycin C is an antitumor antibiotic that inhibits DNA synthesis. Between 39% and 78% of patients with residual tumor have a response to this agent. Side effects include irritative voiding symptoms. A more severe adverse effect is development of rash on the palms and genitalia. Doxorubicin is an antibiotic chemotherapeutic agent associated with a 40% tumor response rate. Local cystitis is a common adverse effect of this medication.

Recurrence of bladder tumor is monitored through periodic cystoscopies and urine cytopathology. If the tumor is refractory to intravesical therapy, a radical cystectomy is often suggested. A typical surveillance protocol is shown in Table 8-5.

Muscle-Invasive Tumors

Muscle-invasive tumors are best treated by radical cystectomy and urinary diversion (continent or incontinent). In men this

■ TABLE 8-5 Bladder Tumor Surveillance Protocol	
Time After Bladder Tumor Resection	**Treatment**
First 2 years	Cystoscopy every 3 months, urine cytology, annual IVP
Years 3 and 4	Cystoscopy every 6 months, urine cytology, annual IVP
Years 5 and beyond	Annual cystoscopy, urine cytology, and IVP

IVP, intravenous pyelography.

procedure involves removal of the bladder and prostate, whereas in women it involves removal of the bladder and uterus and can include resection of the vaginal wall and urethra for tumors that invade the bladder neck.

A bilateral pelvic lymph node dissection is usually performed simultaneously with radical cystectomy. Lymph node metastases are identified in approximately 20% to 35% of patients. Patients with lymph node metastases have a poorer prognosis, although cystectomy and lymphadenectomy can be curative in up to 33% of patients with limited disease.

Additional therapies for muscle-invasive bladder cancer include radiotherapy and chemotherapy. Radiotherapy is an alternative to cystectomy in patients with deeply invasive disease. Approximately 15% of patients have bowel or bladder complications from radiation. The 5-year survival rates for advanced bladder cancer treated with radiation are 20% to 40%. Chemotherapy can be given by single or multiple agents. The most effective single agent is cisplatin, whereas multiagent therapy utilizes methotrexate, vinblastine, doxorubicin (Adriamycin), and cyclophosphamide. Approximately 20% to 30% of patients receiving multidrug regimens achieve a complete response at 1 year. Treatment is associated with significant toxicities, including death in 3% of patients.

Prostate Cancer

■ Epidemiology

Prostate cancer is the most common malignancy diagnosed in men in the United States. Estimates indicate that 1 in 10 men will develop prostate cancer in their lifetime. The incidence of prostate cancer increases with age. The mean age at diagnosis is 65 years, and prostate cancer is rare in men younger than 50. In fact, the probability of prostate cancer developing in a man younger than 40 is approximately 1 in 10,000.

■ **Risk Factors**

Blacks have a higher risk of developing prostate cancer and have a higher mortality rate from the disease than the white population. Having a family history of a first-degree relative with prostate cancer carries a twofold increase in risk. High fat consumption is a possible risk factor. Diets low in animal fat and protein decrease the risk. In addition, certain foods may offer some protection, including vitamin E, selenium, and lycopene from tomato-based foods.

■ **Pathology**

Most carcinomas of the prostate are adenocarcinomas (>95%). About 4% of cases have transitional cell morphology and are thought to arise from the urothelial lining of the prostatic urethra. Other infrequent types include neuroendocrine carcinomas or sarcomas. Approximately 70% of adenocarcinomas develop in the peripheral zone of the prostate, 20% in the transition zone, and 10% in the central zone.

The Gleason grading system is a histologic grade of 1 to 5 and is based on the pattern of glandular architecture and cells visualized under lower-power microscope. The sum of the most predominant grade and the second most common pattern determines the Gleason score. A Gleason score of 4 is a well-differentiated tumor with a good prognosis, whereas a score of 8 to 9 represents a poorly differentiated tumor and has a poor prognosis.

Prostatic intraepithelial neoplasia (PIN) is a dysplastic lesion histologically characterized by loss of cellular polarity and pleomorphism, and is considered to be a premalignant lesion or carcinoma in situ. PIN is classified into two categories: low grade and high grade. Eighty percent of high-grade PIN, in contrast to 20% of low-grade PIN, are associated with invasive prostate cancer. Staging of prostate cancer is based on the TNM system, as outlined in Table 8-6.

The spread of prostate cancer to the lymph nodes includes the obturator nodal packet and from there to the common iliac and para-aortic lymph nodes. The usual sites for metastases from prostate cancer are the lymph nodes, bones, and lungs. Skeletal metastases are common in advanced prostate cancer.

■ **Clinical Manifestations**

Signs and Symptoms

Current screening recommendations by the American Urological Association (AUA) are that both prostate-specific antigen (PSA) testing and digital rectal examination (DRE) should be offered annually to men beginning at age 50. Younger men who are at

■ **TABLE 8-6 TNM System for Prostate Cancer**

Stage	Characteristics
T1	Nonpalpable tumor found by imaging
T1a	Tumor found at transurethral resection of prostate; 5% or less is cancerous with Gleason score ≤ 7
T1b	Tumor found at transurethral resection of prostate; >5% is cancerous with Gleason score ≥ 7
T2	Palpable tumor confined to the prostate
T2a	Tumor involves one lobe or less
T2b	Tumor involves more than one lobe
T3	Palpable tumor beyond the prostate
T3a	Unilateral extracapsular extension
T3b	Bilateral extracapsular extension
T3c	Tumor invades seminal vesicles
T4	Tumor is fixed or invades adjacent structures
T4a	Tumor invades bladder neck, external sphincter, and/or rectum
T4b	Tumor invades levator muscles and/or is fixed to pelvic wall
N0	No lymph node metastasis
N1	Metastasis in single lymph node (<2 cm in diameter)
N2	Metastasis in single lymph node (>2 but <5 cm) or in multiple nodes (<5 cm)
N3	Metastasis in regional lymph nodes >5 cm in diameter
M0	No evidence of distant metastases
M1	Distant metastases

high risk (blacks and those with a family history, particularly in first-degree relatives) should be screened beginning at age 40.

Most often there are no symptoms associated with early-stage prostate cancer. Occasionally, local disease may present with irritative symptoms similar to benign prostatic hyperplasia (nocturia or weakness of stream). Rarely, in advanced disease, skeletal bone pain may be a presenting symptom of bone metastases. Hematospermia is a very rare presenting symptom of prostate cancer.

On DRE, a discrete, hard nodule 0.5 cm or larger is sometimes palpable. It is important to assess the seminal vesicles to determine the extent of local disease. Physical examination findings of adenopathy, lower extremity edema, and bony tenderness may indicate metastatic disease.

■ **Diagnostic Evaluation**

Laboratory Evaluation

Prostate-specific antigen is a serine protease produced by the prostatic epithelium and secreted in the seminal fluid in large quantities.

■ TABLE 8-7 Age-Related Normal Prostate-Specific Antigen Values	
Age (yr)	Normal PSA Level (ng/mL)
40–49	0–2.5
50–59	0–3.5
60–69	0–4.5
70–79	0–6.5

Its function is to liquefy the ejaculate, enabling fertilization. PSA is normally secreted and stored within the ductal system of the prostate. Prostatic disease changes the normal cellular architecture that keeps PSA within the ductal system, altering the serum levels. Serum levels of PSA may be increased by a variety of factors, such as inflammation of the prostate, benign prostatic hyperplasia, prostatic infection, urinary retention, prostate cancer, and bladder catheterization. Studies have shown that DRE causes a subclinical increase in PSA.

To improve the specificity and positive predictive value of the PSA test, PSA velocity, age-adjusted ranges, and PSA forms have been developed. PSA velocity refers to the rate of change of serum PSA levels, and a rapid increase compared with normal values has been shown to correlate with a higher risk of developing cancer. It is thought that PSA levels increase slowly with BPH but more quickly with prostate cancer. Age-adjusted PSA ranges were defined because serum PSA levels increase with age. These age-adjusted ranges increase the sensitivity of detecting prostate cancer in younger patients and increase the specificity in older patients. Normal age-specific PSA reference range levels are listed in Table 8-7. PSA exists in different forms, the most common being bound to various serum proteins. Free PSA is the proportion of total PSA that is not bound to these proteins. The lower the free PSA level is, the higher the risk of having prostate cancer.

PSA can also be elevated in conditions other than prostate cancer, as indicated in Box 8-1.

■ BOX 8-1 Age-Related Normal Conditions That Can Elevate PSA
Benign prostate hyperplasia
Urinary tract infection
Acute or chronic prostatitis
Urinary retention
Prostate needle biopsy

Imaging Studies

A palpable prostatic nodule or an abnormal elevation in PSA level warrants further evaluation. A transrectal ultrasound (TRUS) is used to examine the prostate for hypoechoic areas, which commonly are associated with prostate cancers but are not specific enough for diagnostic purposes. Usually 6 to 18 systematic biopsies of peripheral and transitional zones are taken, regardless of ultrasonographic abnormalities. Complications include sepsis and bleeding. Prophylactic antibiotics are given prior to the procedure and typically include an oral quinolone taken just before and again 12 hours after the procedure.

Bone scan is helpful in detecting bone metastases and is reserved for high-grade, large-volume tumors, a significant elevation in PSA (>20 ng/mL), or in the presence of bone pain. A chest radiograph can be used as a baseline study or to help detect rare pulmonary metastases in selected cases.

■ Treatment

Management of prostate cancer remains controversial because it is dependent on many factors, such as age, life expectancy, extent of disease, and quality of life. This section briefly discusses some of the options available.

Surgery

Radical prostatectomy involves the complete removal of the prostate, seminal vesicles, and the prostatic urethra. It is the most common form of treatment for organ-confined disease and is offered to younger patients (<70 years) with a better than average life expectancy. Besides common surgical risks, side effects specific to this procedure include impotence (even with nerve-sparing techniques) and total or stress incontinence. Impotence rates range from approximately 10% to 75% depending on several factors such as presurgical erectile function, age, history of radiation status, and intactness of the cavernosal nerves. Patients with organ-confined disease have 10-year disease-free survival rates ranging from 70% to 85%. Those with focal extracapsular extension have a 10-year disease-free survival rate of 75%. Patients with more extensive extracapsular extension have a disease-free survival rate of 40%.

Radiation Therapy

External beam radiotherapy (XRT) is typically a 6-week course of daily treatments. Although short-term data (<5 years) suggest that XRT is comparable to surgery, long-term recurrence and PSA failure rates are much higher than with radical prostatectomy. The advantage of XRT is that it is a noninvasive method of treating prostate cancer. Adverse effects related to external beam radiation therapy include cystitis, proctitis, enteritis, impotence, urinary retention, and incontinence.

Interstitial radiotherapy or brachytherapy is an ultrasound-guided implantation of radioactive seeds, usually containing iodine 125, into the prostate. Brachytherapy is an alternative to radical prostatectomy for local, early-stage disease (PSA <10 ng/mL, Gleason score <6), as seen in short-term studies. The advantage of brachytherapy over XRT is that it potentially allows selective radiation to the prostate and less to the surrounding tissues. Significant side effects include urinary retention, incontinence, and erectile dysfunction.

Cryotherapy

Cryotherapy involves freezing the prostate using multiple probes in a fashion similar to that used with brachytherapy. Studies to date suggest short-term success in terms of negative post-treatment biopsies and a decrease in PSA levels to an undetectable value. The morbidity of this procedure can include irritative voiding symptoms and rectourethral fistula formation. Long-term results of this procedure are not yet known.

Hormonal Therapy

Hormonal therapy is usually reserved for patients who aren't good surgical candidates or in patients with metastatic disease. Normal and cancerous growth of the prostate is under the influence of testosterone and dihydrotestosterone (DHT), an intracellular androgen responsible for prostatic cell growth and development. Primary androgen blockade can be achieved either through a bilateral orchiectomy or with the use of luteinizing hormone-releasing hormone (LHRH) agonists (such as leuprolide) alone or in combinations with antiandrogen agents (flutamide, nilutamide, and bicalutamide). LHRH agonists have no effect on adrenal androgens; therefore, combination with an antiandrogen agent allows for a better response. Antiandrogens competitively bind to the DHT receptor. Controversy still exists regarding the efficacy of combination androgen blockade versus single therapy. Side effects of hormone therapy include hot flashes, gynecomastia, decreased libido, impotence, osteoporosis, and flare phenomenon caused by the surge of LH and FSH. Antiandrogens are sometimes used prior to initiating LHRH therapy to prevent this flare phenomenon.

■ Prognosis

The most important and established prognostic indicators for prostate carcinoma include the Gleason grade, the extent of tumor volume, and the presence of capsular penetration or margin positivity at the time of prostatectomy. Biochemical failure or recurrence is defined by a rise in PSA level to greater than 0.5 ng/mL after initial therapy, which should be confirmed by three consecutive test results, each 6 months apart. Patients are followed on a semiannual or annual basis with a digital rectal examination to evaluate for recurrence (induration) as well as determination of serum PSA level. Bone and CT scans are done on a less frequent basis, such as annually or every other year, depending on the results of the DRE and PSA.

Urethral Cancer

■ Epidemiology

Urethral cancer is a rare cancer, constituting less than 1% of all genitourinary cancers. It is more common in whites than in blacks and usually occurs during the sixth to seventh decades. Urethral cancer is the only genitourinary malignancy that is more common in females than in males, by a ratio of 4:1.

■ Risk Factors

In women, factors such as chronic irritative voiding symptoms, recurrent urinary tract infections, and a history of sexually transmitted diseases are believed to cause chronic inflammation leading to cellular dysplasia. In men, a history of urethral stricture disease and venereal disease is found in a majority of the cases.

■ Pathology

The normal epithelium of the urethra progresses from transitional epithelium to squamous epithelium as it courses distally. Therefore, urethral tumors are mostly squamous cell carcinomas (80%), followed by transitional cell carcinoma (15%) and adenocarcinomas (<5%). In females, the most common sites of tumor invasion are the labia, vagina, and bladder neck. In males, most lesions occur primarily in the bulbomembranous and penile regions. Urethral cancer metastasizes to the pelvic and inguinal nodes. Staging is by the TNM system.

■ Clinical Manifestations

Signs and Symptoms
Unfortunately, presentation is often late due to the insidious nature of this disease, and patients often have metastatic disease. Because the signs and symptoms are nonspecific, the diagnosis may often take quite some time because of misdiagnoses and failure of the patient to seek medical consultation. Patients usually present with painless initial or terminal hematuria or with frank bloody discharge, obstructive voiding symptoms (hesitancy, straining), irritative

voiding symptoms (frequency, urgency, dysuria), and perineal pain. Physical examination reveals a palpable periurethral mass and, less commonly, a perineal abscess or urethrocutaneous fistula.

■ Diagnostic Evaluation

Cystourethroscopy with tissue biopsies is the gold standard for diagnosis. The urethral mucosa appears grossly abnormal and is characterized by erythema, surface ulceration, and papillary growth or fungating mass that bleeds easily within the urethra.

■ Treatment

Surgery is the treatment of choice for male urethral cancer. The extent of surgery depends on the location of the tumor within the urethra and the clinical stage. Low-grade lesions may be treated by transurethral resection (TUR), but require close follow-up evaluation with periodic cystoscopic examinations. High-grade lesions in the distal urethra can be managed by a wide surgical excision or partial penectomy in men. Radiation therapy is an option for women with early or low-grade lesions. Most women require radical cystectomy with urethrectomy due to the proximity of urethral disease to the bladder neck and bladder. Chemotherapy with multiple agents is reserved for metastatic disease.

Penile Cancer

■ Epidemiology

Penile cancer is rare in the United States, but may represent up to 30% of all cancers diagnosed in men living in Asia, Africa, or South America. It is rare before the age of 40, with most cases occurring in the seventh decade.

■ Risk Factors

Penile cancer is almost nonexistent in areas where circumcision is practiced, especially when it is done at the neonatal age. It is theorized that chronic irritation from smegma, poor hygiene, and balanitis might be contributory. The human papilloma virus (HPV) types 16, 18, and 21 and the herpes virus have also been implicated in the development of penile cancer. In addition, certain premalignant lesions associated with penile cancer include leukoplakia, balanitis xerotica obliterans, and giant condyloma acuminata (Buschke-Löwenstein tumor).

■ Pathology

Most (95%) of penile cancers are squamous cell carcinomas. Occasionally, basal cell carcinomas, melanomas, and sarcoma

(including Kaposi's sarcoma) occur. Carcinoma in situ is characterized by two different disease processes. Bowen's disease is a
squamous cell carcinoma in situ that appears as an erythematous
plaque, usually on the penile shaft. Erythroplasia of Queyrat is a
velvety, erythematous lesion that involves the glans. These lesions
typically start on the glans or foreskin and gradually grow laterally along the surface, eventually covering the entire glans and pre-
puce and ultimately invading the corpora of the penis. Tumor
spread follows the lymphatic drainage, initially into the superficial inguinal nodes, then to the deep inguinal nodes, and finally
into the pelvic nodes.

■ Clinical Manifestations

Signs and Symptoms
The most common presenting symptom is a nonhealing penile
lesion. Other presenting signs may include ulcerations, erythema,
induration, and a history of inability to retract the foreskin. On
physical examination, it is important to assess inguinal lymph
node status (normal or palpable lymph nodes).

■ Treatment

Partial or total penectomy with a wide negative margin is the
first-line treatment of penile cancer, regardless of inguinal node
status. If the patient has palpable inguinal nodes, broad-spectrum
antibiotic therapy (penicillin derivatives or cephalosporins) for
6 weeks is necessary to reduce nodal inflammation. If lymph
nodes do not regress, then an inguinal lymph node dissection is
necessary. In patients with no palpable lymph nodes, a close follow-up is indicated because lymph node involvement worsens
the prognosis, reducing the 5-year survival rate to 20% to 50%.
However, in patients with higher-stage disease that invades the
corpora cavernosa, inguinal lymph node dissection is performed
regardless of whether the nodes are palpable. The incidence of
lymph node metastasis is approximately 50% when the corpora
is invaded by cancer.

Radiation therapy is an alternative to surgery for a select few
patients that have a small (< 3 cm) superficial, noninvasive lesion
on the glans or coronal sulcus. The advantage of radiation therapy is that the patient can remain potent. Other candidates are
those who refuse surgery or who have metastatic disease and need
some form of palliative therapy.

Testicular Tumors

Although testicular cancer is rare, it is the most common malignancy in males aged 15 to 35 years. Classification is based on the

■ TABLE 8-8 Testicular Tumor and the Peak Age of Occurrence	
Tumor	**Age (yr)**
Yolk sac tumors	Infants and boys
Choriocarcinoma	20–30
Teratoma	25–30
Embryonal	25–30
Seminoma	35–45
Malignant lymphomas	>50

histologic type and is important in determining appropriate therapy. The two major divisions are germ cell and non–germ cell tumors. Germ cell tumors can be further divided into seminomas and nonseminomatous germ cell tumors (NSGCT), which include embryonal cell carcinomas, teratomas, and choriocarcinoma. Non–germ cell tumors include gonadoblastomas and tumors derived from Leydig and Sertoli cells.

■ **Epidemiology**

More than 7000 cases of germ cell tumors are diagnosed each year, with an overall lifetime risk of 1 in 500. The most common age group affected is those from 20 to 45 years; specific subtypes of cancers are more prevalent in certain age groups (Table 8-8). The incidence of testicular cancer in whites is four times greater than that of the black population. Interestingly, testicular cancer is more common on the right side, which correlates with a higher incidence of undescended testis on the same side.

■ **Risk Factors**

There is no definitive cause of testicular cancer, although a well-established link between undescended testis and testicular cancer exists. In fact, nearly 10% of the testicular cancer cases have a history of testicular maldescent. The risk of developing testicular cancer in a male with a history of cryptorchid testis is 5- to 15-fold higher than in those with normally descended testes. Risk is greater for the abdominal versus inguinal location of an undescended testis. Orchidopexy does not prevent tumor formation, but may reduce the risk if done prior to puberty (<8 years). Another advantage of this procedure is that it allows for easier examination of the testes in the future. There is no relationship between testicular trauma and subsequent development of testicular cancer, although trauma to the area may bring attention to a pre-existing mass.

■ BOX 8-2 Types and Incidences of Testicular Cancer

Mixed germ cell tumor (40%)
Seminoma (35%)
Embryonal cell carcinoma (20%)
Teratoma (5%)
Choriocarcinoma (1%)

■ Pathology

Germ Cell Tumors

The pathology of testicular tumors involves mutation of a totipotential germ cell into seminoma or nonseminoma. The process of further differentiation includes extra- and intraembryonic differentiation. Box 8-2 presents the incidence of the pathologic types of testicular cancers.

Seminomas

Seminomas are the most common testicular cancer. They arise from the seminiferous epithelium and are composed of sheets of large round cells with clear cytoplasm. There are three histologic variants of pure seminomas: classic, anaplastic, and spermatocytic. Anaplastic seminoma is characterized by increased mitotic activity compared with the classic type. Spermatocytic seminoma is characterized by cells resembling maturing spermatogonia and is an indolent tumor that rarely metastasizes.

Nonseminomatous Tumors

EMBRYONAL CARCINOMA. Embryonal carcinomas are characterized by a small gray-white lesion with irregular margins causing extensive hemorrhage and necrosis. They are more aggressive than seminomas, with more than 60% presenting with metastases at the time of initial presentation.

TERATOMA. Teratomas arise from primitive totipotential germ cells and therefore may contain derivatives of all three cell layers: ectoderm, endoderm, and mesoderm. The tumor may be cystic or solid with areas of hemorrhage and necrosis and may contain a wide variety of tissue types, such as bone, teeth, muscle, and cartilage. This is the least aggressive form of testicular cancer.

CHORIOCARCINOMA. Choriocarcinoma is the most aggressive of the NSGCTs. It metastasizes hematogenously to lungs, liver, brain, and other viscera very early in the disease process. Pure testicular choriocarcinomas are rare, but are often a component of mixed germ cell tumors. Both syncytiotrophoblasts and cytotrophoblasts need to be present for diagnosis.

YOLK SAC TUMOR. Yolk sac tumors, although generally rare, are the most common pediatric testis tumor. Median age at diagnosis is 24 months. The presence of eosinophilic PAS-positive inclusions in the cytoplasm of clear cells on histologic examination provides the definitive diagnosis.

Nonseminomatous–Germ Cell Tumors

Non–germ cell tumors are most commonly derived from the interstitial cells (Leydig cells). In addition, the supporting cells (Sertoli cells) and gonadoblastoma constitute the remaining small percentage in this group.

Other secondary tumors, such as lymphoma, leukemia, and metastatic tumors, are very rare. Lymphoma is most commonly diagnosed in older men (>50 years) and may present as a late manifestation of advanced lymphoma or as an initial presentation of an occult disease. The histologic type most commonly seen on examination reveals a diffuse histiocytic lymphoma. Leukemic infiltration of the testis is common in children with relapse of acute lymphocytic leukemia. Finally, metastasis to the testis is primarily from the prostate.

■ Clinical Manifestations

Signs and Symptoms
The most common presenting symptom is a painless testicular mass, either reported by the patient or incidentally found on physical examination. Associated symptoms may also include a feeling of dull ache or heaviness in the lower abdomen. In some patients, acute scrotal pain and swelling may occur due to intra-tumoral hemorrhage and necrosis and is sometimes confused with epididymitis or testicular torsion. Symptoms of advanced disease include weight loss, cough, and back or bone pain.

Examination should begin with palpation of the normal testis and evaluation for size, consistency, texture, mobility, nodule, or mass. Physical examination usually confirms the presence of a firm testicular lump. A coexisting hydrocele may obscure underlying malignancy, and an ultrasound is helpful for complete evaluation. A full examination is necessary to evaluate for lymphadenopathy, pleural effusion, abdominal mass, hepatomegaly, and lower limb edema, which are suggestive of advanced disease. Gynecomastia may be present and is secondary to tumor estradiol production.

■ Diagnostic Evaluation

Laboratory Testing
Testing for the serum tumor markers α-fetoprotein (AFP), β-human chorionic gonadotropin (β-hCG), and lactate dehydrogenase (LDH)

is necessary in the complete workup of a patient suspected of testicular cancer. This allows for determining diagnosis, staging, prognosis, and response to therapy. AFP is produced by yolk sac cells and is elevated in nonseminomatous tumors, specifically embryonal carcinomas, teratomas, and yolk sac tumors. A histologic diagnosis of pure seminoma indicates an undetected nonseminomatous tumor component. β-hCG is produced by syncytiotrophoblastic tissue, and increased levels are found in all choriocarcinomas. In addition, increased levels are seen in some embryonal cell tumors and pure seminomas. Elevated LDH levels are not specific for testicular tumors, but are useful in correlating tumor burden in NSGCTs and advanced seminomas.

Imaging Studies

Scrotal ultrasound is usually the first step after a complete physical examination to evaluate the architecture of the testis. US can detect testicular masses and help distinguish between extra- and intratesticular masses. After the diagnosis of testicular cancer, chest radiographs and CT scans are used in the clinical staging of the disease. This is important in determining the appropriate adjunctive radiotherapy and chemotherapy. Staging of testicular cancer is displayed in Table 8-9.

■ Treatment

In patients with an acute onset of pain in whom epididymitis is suspected or who have no palpable mass, a trial of antibiotics is reasonable, since infectious epididymitis or orchitis is more common than tumor. A testicular US is indicated if symptoms and signs are not controlled or do not improve within 2 weeks.

Surgery

A radical inguinal orchiectomy is the procedure of choice for definitive diagnosis and treatment. A transscrotal or preoperative testicular biopsy is contraindicated because of the possibility of metastases to the scrotal lymphatic drainage.

■ TABLE 8-9 Staging of Testicular Cancer	
Stage	**Characteristics**
I	Limited to the testis, epididymis, and spermatic cord
II	Limited to retroperitoneal lymph nodes below the diaphragm
IIA	Nodes <2 cm in diameter
IIB	Nodes 2–5 cm in diameter
IIC	Nodes >5 cm in diameter
III	Metastatic to supradiaphragmatic nodal or visceral sites

Adjunctive Therapy

If clinical staging or tumor markers remain elevated after a radical orchiectomy, systemic disease should be suspected, and adjuvant therapy is then recommended. Seminomas are very sensitive to radiation, which is the treatment of choice in early, small-volume disease. Platinum-based chemotherapy (such as bleomycin, etoposide, and cisplatin) is used for bulky or advanced metastatic disease. Nonseminomas are less sensitive to radiation but are highly responsive to platinum-based chemotherapy. If para-aortic lymph nodes remain enlarged after chemotherapy and radiotherapy, a retroperitoneal lymph node dissection (RPLND) may be curative. This procedure involves removing the lymph nodes where testicular carcinoma is likely to occur. On the right side, dissection will involve the interaortocaval nodal system, whereas on the left side, dissection will involve the para-aortic nodal system. This procedure carries a high risk of subsequent ejaculatory and erectile dysfunction due to the interruption of sympathetic nerve fibers of the pelvis.

■ **Prognosis**

With refinements in surgery and chemotherapy and radiotherapy protocols, survival in testicular cancer has dramatically improved. Table 8-10 displays approximate 5-year disease-free survival rates based on stage and treatment.

■ **TABLE 8-10 Survival Rates for Testicular Cancer Based on Stage**

Stage and Type	Treatment	Five-Year Disease-Free Survival (%)
Seminoma		
I	Orchiectomy + XRT	98
IIa	Orchiectomy + XRT	92–94
IIb and higher	Orchiectomy + chemotherapy	35–75
NSGCT		
I	Orchiectomy + RPLND	96–100
IIb	Orchiectomy + chemotherapy	90
IIc and higher	Orchiectomy + chemotherapy	55–80

XRT, external beam radiotherapy; NSGCT, nonseminomatous germ cell tumors; RPLND, retroperitoneal lymph node dissection.

Non–Germ Cell Tumors of the Testis

■ Leydig Cell Tumors

Leydig cell tumors are the most common non–germ cell tumors of the testis and account for 3% of all testicular tumors. They are common in two age groups: between 5 and 9 years and between 25 and 35 years. Approximately 25% occur in childhood. Physical findings include gynecomastia and virilization. Laboratory findings include elevated serum and urine 17 ketosteroids and estrogen. Radical orchiectomy is the initial treatment for these patients. RPLND is recommended for malignant lesions, which are heralded by elevations of 17 ketosteroids to approximately 30 times the normal values.

■ Sertoli Cell Tumors

Sertoli cell tumors account for 1% of all testicular tumors. They are common in two age groups: younger than 1 year, and between 20 and 45 years. Approximately 10% of the lesions are malignant. Physical findings include the presence of a testicular mass, virilization, and gynecomastia. Radical orchiectomy is the treatment of choice. RPLND is indicated for the presence of malignancy. The roles of radiotherapy and chemotherapy are not well defined.

9 Genitourinary Trauma

Renal Trauma

■ Pathogenesis

Renal trauma represents the most common of all urologic injuries and is often associated with other abdominal organ injuries. Although injuries to the cardiopulmonary organs take precedence in an unstable patient, renal trauma needs to be assessed on a secondary survey because it may have a subtle presentation. Blunt renal trauma accounts for 75% to 85% of all renal injuries; the remainder are due to penetrating renal injuries. Penetrating injuries include gunshots and stab wounds, whereas common blunt traumas include motor vehicle accidents and sports-related injuries. In blunt trauma, the kidney sustains injury by being crushed between the anterior ends of the lower ribs and the upper lumbar vertebrae. Therefore, fracture of the lower ribs and ecchymosis of the flank may provide clues to underlying renal injuries.

■ Clinical Manifestations

Signs and Symptoms

Hematuria (gross or microscopic) and the presence of shock (systolic blood pressure <90 mm Hg) are important determinants that further evaluation will be required in patients with renal trauma. General and complete physical examination is a part of any major trauma. For renal trauma specifically, examine for flank contusions and for abdominal or flank tenderness. Absent bowel sounds may indicate severe intra-abdominal injury or a retroperitoneal hematoma-induced paralytic ileus.

■ Diagnostic Evaluation

Laboratory Studies

Gross hematuria or microhematuria is usually present in most renal trauma. The degree of hematuria does not correlate with the extent of injury, because significant renal injury may also be present in the absence of hematuria. This is commonly seen in renal pedicle injuries that result in arterial damage, causing ischemic injury that does not result in bleeding.

■ TABLE 9-1 American Association of Trauma's Surgery Staging of Renal Trauma

Minor

Grade I	Hematuria, contusion, subcapsular hematoma, intact renal capsule
Grade II	Minor cortical laceration, or nonexpanding perirenal hematoma

Major

Grade III	Major laceration into cortex and medulla but without extravasation
Grade IV	Major laceration into cortex, medulla, and collecting system
Grade V	Multiple major lacerations (shattered kidney) or renal pedicle avulsion.

Imaging Studies

Imaging studies are necessary to define the extent of renal trauma and to aid in the determination of appropriate management. Ultrasonography is limited in the initial workup because it does not evaluate renal function, and it cannot distinguish hematoma from urinary extravasation. A contrast-enhanced helical computed tomographic (CT) scan is the preferred test in the evaluation of significant upper tract blunt or penetrating renal trauma. CT helps in visualizing parenchymal lacerations and urinary extravasation, in addition to delineating other intra-abdominal injuries. Table 9-1 presents the American Association of Trauma's staging system.

■ Treatment

Most blunt renal trauma can be managed conservatively with complete bed rest and sedation. Urinary extravasation requires antibiotic administration because such fluid can contain both blood and urine when the collecting system is disrupted. Broad-spectrum agents such as ampicillin and gentamicin are typically used in this situation. Large fluid collections may require percutaneous drainage.

Most penetrating injuries are serious and require surgical intervention. Absolute indications for surgical intervention are listed in Box 9-1. Minor urinary extravasation can usually be treated conservatively until it spontaneously resolves, or can be treated by

■ BOX 9-1 Absolute Indications for Surgery for Renal Trauma

Penetrating renal injuries
Renal pedicle or other arterial injury
Urinary extravasation on intravenous pyelography
Retroperitoneal hematoma with progressive blood loss

placing a ureteral stent to assist with urinary drainage. Long-term follow-up is necessary because hypertension, arteriovenous fistula, and pyelonephritis are late complications of renal trauma.

Injuries to the Ureter

■ Pathogenesis

Ureteral injuries are relatively uncommon because the retroperitoneal location of the ureter confers some protection from external trauma. The most common cause of injury to the ureter is iatrogenic during intra-abdominal and pelvic surgery, such as colorectal surgery and hysterectomy. This is because of the ureter's close relation to the pelvic vessels, the broad ligament, and the uterine artery. Blunt trauma causing injury to the ureter is also uncommon when compared with penetrating injuries. In pelvic fractures, the ureter is most likely to be injured as it crosses the pelvic brim.

■ Clinical Manifestations

Signs and Symptoms

Blunt ureteral injury usually presents with hematuria and flank pain similar to that seen with renal colic. Postoperative ureteral injury usually presents with fever, flank pain, paralytic ileus with nausea and vomiting, or drainage from the surgical wound or drain. Bilateral ureteral injury will result in anuria.

Physical examination may reveal abdominal distention, abdominal tenderness, and a palpable mass indicating the presence of urinoma.

■ Diagnostic Evaluation

Laboratory Studies

Serum creatinine level is often elevated due to extravasation and reabsorption of urine or with bilateral ureteral injury. Urinalysis usually reveals microscopic hematuria with ureteral contusion or partial ureteral tear, but hematuria is rarely present in cases of complete ureteral transection. Fluid from drains placed from prior surgical procedures can be sent for creatinine level analysis to help determine its origin. As mentioned, this injury can occur after a difficult hysterectomy or colon resection in the presence of significant inflammation. A creatinine level near normal indicates that the fluid drainage is lymph, whereas a urine sample will have a much higher creatinine level.

Imaging Studies

An intravenous pyelogram (IVP) is the initial radiographic test of choice in a suspected ureteric injury. Findings include hydronephrosis of the affected kidney, delayed excretion of the contrast, and absence of the contrast below the level of the injury. In a complete transaction, the urine may drain freely into the abdomen or retroperitoneum. Cystoscopy with retrograde ureterography can also be performed to evaluate ureteral injuries. This procedure may also be therapeutic, as will be discussed shortly.

■ Treatment

The treatment of choice depends on the location and the severity of the ureteric injury. In general, minor injuries with minimal extravasation can be managed conservatively by placing a ureteral stent for 3 to 4 weeks. In patients with significant injuries, open surgical repair may be required. If possible, a tension-free primary anastomosis is preferred. In cases where reanastomosis cannot be done in a tension-free fashion, various surgical techniques such as a Boari flap may be used. The **Boari bladder flap** involves tubularization of a flap of bladder to create additional length so that the ureter can be implanted directly into the bladder.

Injuries to the Bladder

■ Pathogenesis

The bladder lies extraperitoneally in the space of Retzius within the bony pelvis. The mechanism of bladder injury depends on whether the bladder was empty or full at the time of trauma. When full, the bladder can assume an intra-abdominal position by pushing against the peritoneal reflection on the dome. Therefore, a direct blow or a penetrating injury to the lower abdomen will result in an intraperitoneal rupture because of a laceration to the dome. On the other hand, an empty bladder remains within the bony pelvis; most commonly, an external force causing a pelvic fracture will result in an extraperitoneal rupture. Bony fragments from the pelvic fracture usually perforate the bladder. In fact, 8% to 10% of all pelvic fractures have an associated bladder injury.

■ Clinical Manifestations

Signs and Symptoms

Initially, an intraperitoneal rupture might not present with any symptoms except for the inability to void. Ultimately, as urine is diverted into the peritoneal cavity, an acute abdomen may develop, with a possible development of a deep pelvic abscess and inflammation. Unlike an intraperitoneal bladder rupture, extravasation from an extraperitoneal rupture may cause suprapubic pain, swelling, and induration from blood and urine tracking up the anterior wall between the transversalis fascia and the peritoneum.

■ Diagnostic Evaluation

Laboratory Studies

Similar to other genitourinary trauma, microscopic or gross hematuria is usually found in most cases of bladder trauma. In addition, an elevation in serum creatinine level is usually seen with intraperitoneal rupture.

Imaging Studies

A cystogram is the radiographic imaging study of choice when evaluating bladder trauma. The bladder should be adequately distended with at least 350 mL of water-soluble contrast in a retrograde fashion through a urethral catheter. It is necessary to take postdrainage films because the contrast may obscure a small leak. If the urethral catheter cannot be passed into the bladder, then a suprapubic catheter can be placed to obtain a cystogram.

■ Treatment

In general, extraperitoneal perforations spontaneously heal within 10 to 14 days. It is important to assist bladder drainage by maintaining the urinary catheter during this time period. Intraperitoneal perforations require surgical exploration and repair.

Injuries to the Urethra

Urethral trauma is categorized by the location of the injury in the anterior or posterior urethra. The anatomical landmark is the urogenital diaphragm, which divides the anterior (bulbous and pendulous) urethra from the posterior (membranous and prostatic) urethra. Traumas of the female urethra are very rare. The mechanisms of injury to the anterior and posterior urethra are different. Anterior urethral injury usually results from straddle injuries (e.g., hitting the crossbar of a bicycle), direct blows to the perineum, or instrumentation (cystoscopy or catheterization). Posterior urethral injury, on the other hand, results from massive injury such as pelvic fractures, which cause the membranous urethra to detach from the bulbous urethra.

■ Clinical Manifestations

Signs and Symptoms

Blood at the external urethral meatus or a bloody urethral discharge is a classic finding in urethral trauma. On physical examination, an anterior urethral injury that is confined by the Buck's fascia will have a "sleeve of penis" injury in which penile bruising and swelling is confined to the penile shaft. If Buck's fascia is ruptured, then the bruising is confined by the next most superficial layer, Colles' fascia, and will result in the characteristic butterfly pattern of ecchymosis. Because Colles' fascia extends up to the clavicles, as does Scarpa's fascia, severe bleeding from an anterior urethral injury might extend up the chest to the clavicles.

A rectal examination is necessary to evaluate sphincter tone and the position of the prostate. A large pelvic hematoma resulting from a pelvic fracture can displace the prostate superiorly. Digital rectal examination may reveal a high-riding, boggy, and ballotable prostate gland.

A Foley catheter should never be introduced in a patient with suspected urethral trauma, especially when gross blood is present at the urethral meatus. The catheter should never be forced against resistance in a patient with perineal trauma because it may convert a partial tear into a complete disruption. Therefore, imaging studies, such as a retrograde urethrography, should be obtained first.

Imaging Studies

Retrograde urethrography is the study of choice when evaluating urethral injury. Free extravasation of contrast is seen at the site of the urethral tear. If no extravasation is seen, and if other genitourinary tract injuries have been ruled out, a patient with a bloody urethral meatus is said to have a urethral contusion.

■ Treatment

Urethral contusion can be managed conservatively by placing a urethral catheter if the patient has difficulty voiding. If complete anterior rupture is indicated on imaging studies, then a cystotomy tube can be placed percutaneously, allowing the urine to be diverted while the urethral laceration heals. A voiding study through the tube can be done later and the length of urethral injury reassessed. Repair of the stricture can be performed at a later date.

In a posterior urethral injury, either a suprapubic catheter is placed without any further surgery or the patient undergoes immediate urethral realignment. In the first option, a suprapubic tube is placed to provide urinary drainage. Cystography is performed 3 months later to assess the length of disruption. Realignment surgery can occur at this time. The second option is immediate urethral realignment. This surgery can be challenging because of persistent bleeding and surrounding hematoma. The incidence of stricture, impotence, and incontinence seems to be higher with this approach.

Pediatric Urology

Ureteropelvic Junction Obstruction

■ Pathogenesis

Congenital anomalies are the most common cause of ureteropelvic junction (UPJ) obstruction. Intrinsic causes can include aperistaltic ureteral segments, stenosis, or valvelike folds. Extrinsic etiology ranges from neoplasms, ureteral kinks, and kidney stones to inflammatory processes.

Regardless of the cause, impediment to flow leads to increased intraluminal hydrostatic pressure, decreased glomerular filtration rate, and finally, impaired tubular function. Baseline intraluminal pressures range from 0 to 5 cm H_2O, whereas pressures during obstruction may exceed 22 cm H_2O. Hydronephrosis is a direct result of this increase in pressure. In fact, UPJ obstruction is the primary cause of hydronephrosis in the pediatric population. Diminished tubular function has a variety of consequences. It may manifest as a decreased ability of the nephron to concentrate urine, an increased urinary sodium concentration, or a reduction in urinary acidification. A differential diagnosis of hydronephrosis is provided in Box 10-1.

■ Epidemiology

UPJ obstruction occurs in 1 in 1500 births, with a male-to-female ratio of 2:1. The majority of cases are unilateral, and there is a slight predominance for the left side.

■ Risk Factors

Associated conditions include multicystic dysplastic kidney, duplication, congenital heart disease, and the VATER syndrome

---

■ BOX 10-1 Differential Diagnosis of Hydronephrosis

Ureteropelvic junction obstruction
Vesicoureteral reflux
Ureterovesical junction obstruction
Megaureter
Multicystic dysplastic kidney

(vertebral anomalies, imperforate anus, tracheoesophageal fistulae, and renal anomalies).

■ Clinical Manifestations

History
Children and infants with UPJ obstruction may present with abdominal masses, gastrointestinal discomfort, hematuria, urinary tract infections, kidney stones, or failure to thrive.

■ Diagnostic Evaluation

Diagnostic tools for UPJ obstruction include ultrasound, diuretic renography, and the Whitaker test, an invasive test that measures the pressure differential between the renal pelvis and the bladder. Pressures above 20 cm H_2O suggest obstruction. Ultrasound is typically the initial investigative test (accuracy of 77%) and usually reveals dilatation of the renal pelvis and nonvisualization of the ureter. Ultrasound may detect obstruction in utero as early as 15 gestational weeks.

■ Treatment

Treatment includes open pyeloplasty and endoscopic endopyelotomy. Both techniques may involve placement of a stent to decompress the kidney. Open correction has a success rate of 95%; surgical approaches can be transperitoneal, anterior extraperitoneal, flank, or dorsal lumbotomy.

Vesicoureteral Reflux

■ Pathogenesis

The typical anatomy of the ureters and bladder is protective against reflux. The ureters enter the bladder at an oblique angle, and the detrusor muscle is compliant and supportive during filling and voiding. In addition, the ureterotrigonal muscles close the ureteral orifice during detrusor contraction.

Primary reflux occurs when anatomic anomalies result in loss of this protection. Clinical findings include a laterally placed ureteral orifice, a weakened trigone, or a shortened submucosal tunnel. Secondary reflux is typically caused by bladder obstruction (due to kidney stones or neoplasms) and elevated intravesical pressures.

■ Epidemiology

Reflux occurs in 1% to 18% of children, with 85% of cases in females. The incidence is also 10 times more common in whites than blacks.

■ Risk Factors

Risk factors include urinary tract infections (UTIs), UPJ obstruction, and ureteral duplication. Patients who have mothers or siblings with reflux are also at an increased risk. Up to 45% of siblings of an affected child will also have reflux.

■ Clinical Manifestations

History

Newborns and infants may present with vague symptoms such as fever, malaise, or failure to thrive, whereas older children tend to present with symptoms of a UTI. Patients with chronic reflux may have symptoms such as impaired growth, renal insufficiency, and hypertension.

■ Diagnostic Evaluation

A voiding cystourethrogram is necessary in newborns with moderate to severe hydronephrosis, in children younger than 5 years with a documented UTI, in any child with a fever and a UTI, and in any male with a UTI unless he is sexually active or has a past urologic history. Figure 10-1 shows the current grading system for reflux.

A renal ultrasound may be used to detect renal scarring or to confirm a secondary cause, such as obstruction.

■ Treatment

Vesicoureteral reflux resolves spontaneously in many children and is more likely to occur when the diagnosis is made at a younger age.

Pharmaceutical management consists of low-dose suppressive antibiotics given once daily and is recommended for initial treatment of reflux grades I, II, or III. Medical intervention is also acceptable for grade IV reflux in a patient younger than 6 years or with unilateral reflux. Amoxicillin is generally given to infants after 6 weeks of age. Trimethoprim-sulfamethoxazole may also be used.

Surgery is indicated in several situations. Surgical intervention is preferred for persistent reflux despite antibiotic therapy, severe bilateral reflux, reflux due to congenital anomalies, failure of renal growth, or deterioration of renal function. Intravesical, extravesical, and combinational approaches are made with a surgical success rate near 99%. Complications of surgery include persistent reflux and obstruction.

Endoscopic management may also be employed and includes a variety of nonautologous and autologous materials. In either case, the material is positioned behind the ureter to provide additional support and compliance during filling and voiding.

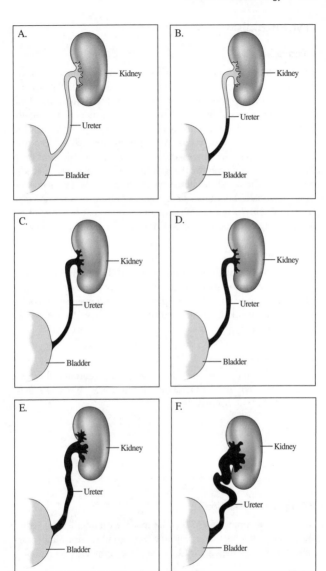

Figure 10-1 • Grading of vesicoureteral reflux. (A) Normal kidney, ureter, and bladder. (B) Grade I vesicoureteral reflux: Urine refluxes part-way up the ureter. (C) Grade II: Urine refluxes all the way up the ureter. (D) Grade III: Urine refluxes all the way up the ureter, with dilatation of the ureter and calyces (part of the kidney where urine collects). (E) Grade IV: Urine refluxes all the way up the ureter with marked dilatation of the ureter and calyces. (F) Grade V: Massive reflux of urine up the ureter, with marked tortuosity and dilatation of the ureter and calyces.

Cryptorchidism

■ Pathogenesis

At 7 weeks' gestation a gene called testis-determining factor on the short arm of chromosome Y begins to regulate the SRY protein. This protein is responsible for the differentiation of the fetal gonad into a testis. Shortly after, the testis begins to secrete testosterone. Testosterone induces the Wolffian duct to form the epididymis and vas deferens. At approximately 36 weeks, the testes, vasa deferentia, and epididymides begin their descent from the level of the kidney to the scrotum. They may arrest at any point along the way, leading to cryptorchidism. The testes may be in an inguinal, abdominal, or ectopic position, or they may be entirely absent. In any case, the cooler environment of the scrotum is ultimately essential for the production of viable spermatozoa.

■ Epidemiology

Undescended testicles occur in 3.4% of full-term infants and in 30% of premature infants, with the majority of cases being unilateral. By 1 year of age, most previously undescended testicles will have descended. Up to 15% of affected boys have a family member with cryptorchidism.

■ Risk Factors

Associated conditions include ambiguous genitalia, hernias, Klinefelter's syndrome, Prader-Willi syndrome, Noonan's syndrome, and cystic fibrosis.

■ Clinical Manifestations

Physical

The physical exam is crucial. Diagnosis is based on physical examination findings, with an accuracy rate of 53% to 84%.

■ Diagnostic Evaluation

An overall accuracy of 44% can be made with a variety of radiologic tools. These include computed tomography, ultrasound, magnetic resonance imaging, testicular arteriography, and venography.

■ Treatment

Treatment for cryptorchidism should be initiated prior to 2 years of age to avoid associated complications. There are two categories of treatment: hormonal and surgical. Hormonal therapy consists of luteinizing hormone-releasing hormone (LHRH) and human chorionic gonadotrophin (hCG). HCG promotes descent by stimulating Leydig cells to produce testosterone. It has an efficacy of between 14% and 50% and is the only hormone approved for the treatment of cryptorchidism in the United States. A trial of hormonal therapy may be acceptable before the age of 2. After 2 years of age, an orchiopexy should be performed.

Surgical intervention may be laparoscopic or via an open abdominal approach. The laparoscopic technique tends to be used when the testis is not palpable. In bilateral cases, both sides should be repaired in the same operation, with one exception: In the case of an extremely high-situated testis, unilateral repair is preferred. Left untreated, undescended testes may result in neoplasia, torsion, hernia, and infertility. Prostheses are available for testes that are not salvageable or were removed surgically.

Bladder Exstrophy

■ Pathogenesis

Bladder exstrophy occurs when the anterior wall of the bladder and the anterior abdominal wall fail to close. This is a consequence of abnormal embryologic development.

The cloacal membrane consists of the endoderm and ectoderm. Mesoderm formation between the two layers leads to the development of the pelvic bones and abdominal muscles. The cloaca then divides into the bladder and rectum. Current theory holds that exstrophy occurs when mesenchymal tissue migrates abnormally between ectodermal and endodermal layers of the cloacal membrane. As a result, abnormal formation of the abdominal wall structures occurs. The rectus muscles tend to be displaced laterally, the posterior wall of the bladder is exposed, and the hips may be rotated laterally. The bladder may range from a tiny patch to a volume of 30 cc.

■ Epidemiology

Bladder exstrophy occurs in 1 in 30,000 births and affects males twice as often as females. The anomaly appears to have a hereditary component, because 1 in 70 children of affected parents will also have exstrophy.

■ Clinical Manifestations

Abnormalities of the abdominal wall structures manifest in a variety of ways. Aside from those already mentioned, males may have a shortened and widened penis, cryptorchidism, or retractile testis. Females may have a hemiclitoris, and the vaginal orifice is usually narrow. Duplications of the vagina or uterus are also not uncommon.

■ Diagnostic Evaluation

Prenatal ultrasound may identify exstrophy by 20 weeks' gestation. Ultrasound will show absence of a bladder, as well as a lower abdominal mass. The distance from the umbilicus to anus may be shortened, because the umbilicus is typically set lower.

■ Treatment

Treatment is surgical closure of the bladder, and prognosis is best if surgery is performed within 48 hours of birth. If bladder capacity proves to be too small, bladder augmentation using various tissues may be employed. Stomach, colon, and small bowel have all been utilized for bladder augmentation. Antibiotic prophylaxis should be administered before surgery. Ampicillin and gentamicin are commonly used.

Following surgery, fewer than 50% of patients will be completely continent, because most patients will have abnormal detrusor function. In addition, fertility rate is lower than that of the average population, although not completely absent. The lower fertility rate may be partially attributable to the increased incidence of retrograde ejaculation in this group.

Testicular Torsion

■ Pathogenesis

Testicular torsion is a pediatric emergency. It occurs when the spermatic cord twists around the blood vessels that support the testicle, thus strangulating the blood supply. Most often this occurs spontaneously. However, trauma to the testicle can sometimes trigger spasms in the muscles that attach the testicle to the spermatic cord. As a result, the spermatic cord moves around the testicle.

Males with a bell clapper deformity are more likely to be affected. This occurs when the normal posterior anchoring of the gubernaculum, epididymis, and testis fails to occur. The testis is then free to rotate within the tunica vaginalis of the scrotum. When the testicle rotates on the axis of the spermatic cord, edema and obstruction of the lymphatics occur. Occlusion of venous and arterial vessels ensues.

■ Epidemiology

One in 4000 males under the age of 25 years will be affected. Over 60% of cases occur between the ages of 12 and 18.

■ **BOX 10-2 Differential Diagnosis of Acute Scrotal Pain**

Testicular torsion
Epididymitis
Torsion of appendix testis or appendix epididymis
Incarcerated inguinal hernia
Testicular tumor
Idiopathic scrotal edema
Acute hydrocele
Henoch-Schönlein purpura
Spermatocele
Varicocele

■ **Clinical Manifestations**

History and Physical Exam

Most patients with torsion will present with a history of sudden onset of scrotal pain, swelling, and erythema. Torsion is the primary cause of acute scrotal swelling in boys under the age of 18. Other patients may complain of nausea, vomiting, diaphoresis, and tachycardia. Often, normal landmarks, such as the epididymis, may not be palpable because of edema. Testicular torsion tends to present unilaterally, and the testicle may be located at a higher position than is normal. The differential diagnosis of acute scrotal pain is displayed in Box 10-2.

■ **Diagnostic Evaluation**

Ultrasound with color-flow Doppler or a radioisotope testis scan can be used to measure testicular blood flow, as well as to rule out other causes of inflammation (Figures 10-2 a&b and 10-3).

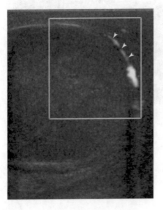

Figure 10-2a • Testicular torsion. Ultrasound of the testis with Doppler flow imaging demonstrates lack of blood flow within the torsed right testis. There is flow peripherally. *(Used with permission of Cedars-Sinai Medical Center, Los Angeles, California.)*

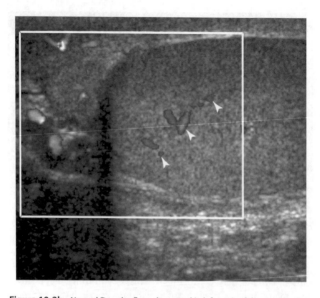

Figure 10-2b • Normal Doppler flow ultrasound in left testis of the same patient as Fig. 10-2a. Arrowheads show areas of blood flow.
(Used with permission of Cedars-Sinai Medical Center, Los Angeles, California.)

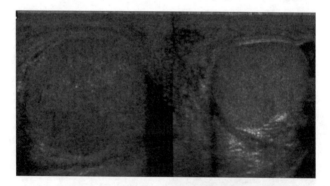

Figure 10-3 • Testicular torsion. Side-by-side comparison with grayscale ultrasound reveals heterogeneous echotexture of the torsed right testis compared to the normal left testis. The patient had the acute onset of pain after falling from a skateboard.
(Used with permission of Cedars-Sinai Medical Center, Los Angeles, California.)

However, the ordering of unnecessary tests may delay prompt surgical intervention, which is crucial.

■ Treatment

Aggressive surgical intervention is necessary because permanent germ cell damage may occur within 4 hours. Testicular salvage is directly influenced by the duration of torsion. If torsion is reversed within 12 hours, the salvage rate approaches 80% to 90%.

If the testis can be untwisted and reveals evidence of good perfusion, as suggested by warmth and a pinkish color, placement of permanent sutures to anchor the testis to the scrotum will prevent further torsion. The contralateral testicle should also be anchored, since the condition may occur on the unaffected side as well. In the absence of normal testicular perfusion, an orchiectomy should be performed.

Hypospadias

Hypospadias is the most common genital abnormality in males, occurring in 1 in 300 of live male births. It occurs when the urethral meatus opens ventrally anywhere between the perineum and the tip of the glans penis. In fact, hypospadias is classified according to the location: glandular, coronal, penile shaft, penoscrotal, or perineal. The most common cases of hypospadias occur at the glans or coronal sulcus. The exact etiology of hypospadias is not known, but it is believed that it results from alterations of the urethral fold closure. Normally, under the influence of testosterone, as the phallus elongates, the urethral folds coalesce in the midline, closing the urethra and forming the median raphe of the scrotum and penis. Therefore, any disruption of testosterone production, such as exogenous estrogen and progestins during gestational age 6 weeks to 9 weeks, may result in hypospadias.

■ Clinical Manifestations

History and Physical Exam

Newborns and infants rarely present with any symptoms, whereas in children and adults the most common complaint is the inability to void with a forward pointing stream. The patient may also complain of an associated downward curvature of the penis with erection (ventral chordee). This is due to an associated hooded foreskin with a deficiency of the ventral skin, shortening of the urethra, and presence of fibrous thickening of the tunica albuginea.

■ Diagnostic Evaluation

A physical examination is adequate to diagnose a hypospadias. Infrequently, it may be associated with other abnormalities such as ambiguous genitalia, making it hard to establish the sex of the child; it is therefore recommended to obtain karyotype in these children. An intravenous pyelogram may also be ordered to exclude any other anomalies of the urinary tract.

■ Treatment

The optimal age for surgical correction is before 2 years of age to avoid cosmetic and fertility problems. A major complication with surgical reconstruction is the formation of a urethrocutaneous fistula, which occurs in 10% of repairs.

1 Common Urologic Consults

Priapism

Priapism is a condition defined by prolonged erection for at least 4 to 6 hours without sexual desire and unrelieved by orgasm. Priapism is considered a urologic emergency.

■ Etiology

Box 11-1 presents some of the common etiologies for priapism. Secondary causes of priapism are classified as either high flow (nonischemic) or low flow (ischemic). High-flow priapism is usually secondary to perineal trauma, whereas low-flow priapism is believed to be a physiologic abnormality in venous drainage. With low-flow priapism, the corpus spongiosum and glans penis are soft and uninvolved. Persistence for several days will lead to interstitial edema and to fibrosis of the corpora cavernosa. The most devastating outcome of priapism is impotence, which is seen in up to 55% of patients.

The antihypertensives most commonly associated with priapism are hydralazine, guanethidine, and prazosin. Antipsychotics include those of the phenothiazine group, of which chlorpromazine is most common, and trazodone. Other phenothiazines implicated in priapism include thioridazine, trifluoperazine, perphenazine, and fluphenazine.

■ BOX 11-1 Etiologies of Priapism

Primary (idiopathic)
Secondary
  Thromboembolic and associated with disease (sickle cell anemia,
    leukemia, fat emboli, pelvic tumors and pelvic infection, malaria,
    and rabies)
  Traumatic (perineal or genital trauma)
  Neurogenic (spinal cord lesions, autonomic neuropathy, and anesthesia)
  Oral medicines and alcohol (antihypertensives, antipsychotics,
    gonadotropin-releasing hormone, cocaine, and heparin)
  Intracavernosal injections for neurogenic or psychogenic impotence
    (papaverine, papaverine with phentolamine, prostaglandin E_1, or
    a mixture of all three)
  Total parenteral nutrition

Spinal and general anesthesia may produce erection during scrub preparation for surgery. Malignancy is thought to cause priapism due to venous drainage obstruction or partial replacement of the sinusoids, which ultimately will cause stasis and thrombosis of the remaining tissue. Similarly, perineal and genital trauma also cause blockage of penile venous drainage due to thrombosis, severe hemorrhage, or tissue edema at the base of the penis.

Total parenteral nutrition has been associated with priapism after infusion of a 20% intravenous fat emulsion (Intralipid). Intralipid is thought to produce its effect by three proposed mechanisms: a direct increase in blood coagulability, adverse effects on cellular components of the blood, and fat emboli.

The most common causes of priapism are idiopathic (46%–60%), alcohol and drug therapy, perineal trauma, and sickle cell disease. Leukemia is the second most common cause of priapism in young boys, following sickle cell anemia.

■ Diagnosis

The diagnosis of priapism is contingent on having a persistent erection for greater than 4 to 6 hours without sexual desire and unrelieved by orgasm. Necessary laboratory studies include a sickle cell preparation for hemoglobin S in all black patients with priapism, complete blood cell count (CBC) to rule out leukemia, a complete drug history, and social history for intracavernosal injections due to impotence. Cavernosal blood gases and duplex ultrasound will differentiate whether the etiology is high-flow (nonischemic) or low-flow (ischemic) priapism. In high-flow priapism, the corporal blood gas values will be similar to arterial blood gases, whereas in low-flow priapism the corporal blood gas values usually show a pH less than 7.25, a PCO_2 greater than 60, and a PO_2 less than 30. A past surgical history may suggest causes related to anesthesia or total parenteral nutrition.

■ Treatment

Treatment is dependent on the results of the history, physical exam, CBC, and cavernosal blood gases. If the etiology of priapism is malignancy, treatment is usually palliative and may include biopsy, oncology consultation, radiation, and chemotherapy for the primary disease.

The initial management of priapism secondary to sickle cell anemia is usually conservative and includes hydration and oxygenation. Hypertransfusion may be effective in those patients who do not respond to hydration and oxygen therapy. In severe instances, corporal irrigation and shunting procedures may be necessary.

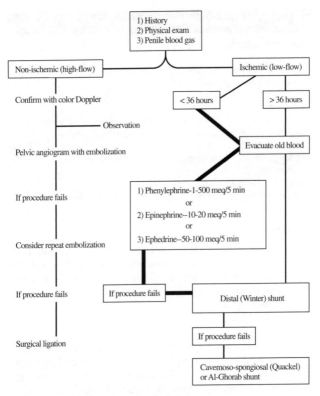

Figure 11-1 • Medical management of priapism.

Anesthesia-induced priapism is treated by inducing deeper anesthesia and may also involve administration of beta blockers, ketamine, or alpha adrenergics.

Figure 11-1 outlines the treatment for high- and low-flow priapism.

Acute Urinary Retention

Acute urinary retention is a sudden inability to urinate that is usually associated with increased urgency, extreme suprapubic pain, and occasional dribbling of small amounts of urine in some cases.

■ **BOX 11-2 Etiology of Acute Urinary Retention**

Benign prostatic hyperplasia
Urethral stricture
Blood clots (status post-transurethral resection procedures of the prostate or bladder)
Bladder neck contracture (postsurgical scarring)
Prostate cancer
Detrusor myopathy (postsurgical recovery from anesthesia)
Neuropathic bladder (trauma, tumor, tabes dorsalis, spina bifida, meningomyelocele)
Drugs (alpha agonists, anticholinergics, antihistamines, anesthetics, antidepressants)
Psychogenic retention
Neurologic disease (multiple sclerosis, Parkinson's disease, amyotrophic
   lateral sclerosis)
Pain (nociceptive retention)

■ **Etiology**

The etiology of acute urinary retention is shown in Box 11-2. Acute urinary retention most commonly occurs in those patients who already have some degree of bladder neck or outlet obstruction. Benign prostatic hyperplasia is the most common cause of acute urinary retention.

■ **Diagnosis**

The diagnosis of acute urinary retention requires a careful history and physical exam looking for a prior history of problems with voiding, urinary retention, urologic surgeries such as transurethral resection of the bladder or prostate, medications, overflow incontinence, and strictures. A digital rectal exam should be done to assess prostate size. Although significant suprapubic pain and a history of not being able to void may be suggestive of acute urinary retention, suprapubic pain may be caused by cystitis or constipation.

■ **Treatment**

The goal of treating acute urinary retention is to use the least invasive technique to reach the outcome of complete urinary drainage Figure 11-2 shows a flowchart for treatment of acute urinary retention.

Fournier's Gangrene

Fournier's gangrene is necrotizing fasciitis of the perineum or genital area. The condition is most commonly seen in men older than 50, yet the mean age of occurrence is 20 to 50 years. Mortality rates for this disease are as high as 50%. Other risk factors are associated with this disease and will be discussed later.

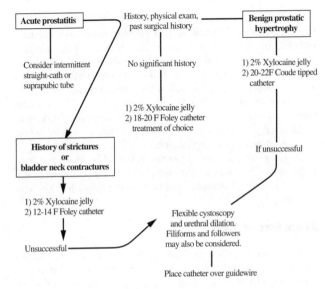

Figure 11-2 • Treatment flowchart for acute urinary retention.

■ Etiology

Fournier's gangrene is secondary to some type of perineal or genital trauma, infection, or surgical incision. These skin defects allow entrance of the bacterial species that cause this disease. Most commonly the bacterial species involved are staphylococci, streptococci, Enterobacteriaceae, *Clostridium*, and *Bacteroides*. The bacterial source for these species is usually the gastrointestinal or genitourinary tract. The etiology is often unknown.

■ Diagnosis

Diagnosis of Fournier's gangrene requires a high index of suspicion and early treatment. Patients at higher risk include those who suffer from diabetes, morbid obesity, immunosuppression, or alcohol abuse or those who take steroid medications. These patients will present with severe perineal or genital pain. Patients may develop fever or chills secondary to necrotizing fasciitis. Necessary laboratory tests include creatinine, electrolytes, arterial blood gases, and hematologic and coagulation studies. Urine, blood, and tissue cultures are required. An abdominal plain film radiograph is also recommended.

■ Treatment

Prompt diagnosis is critical, and differentiation between cellulitis and necrotizing fasciitis may be difficult because of the similarity of symptoms; marked systemic toxicity, however, should be an indicator of necrotizing fasciitis. Yellow or purpuric fluid in a blister overlying the area of suspicion is pathognomonic.

Treatment should begin with intravenous hydration and triple-antibiotic therapy for preparation of surgical débridement of the site. A recommended regimen is gentamicin, metronidazole, and a third-generation cephalosporin such as ceftriaxone.

Postsurgically, the area of excision should be bandaged with gauze soaked in Dakin's solution and changed several times daily. Antibiotic therapy should continue until granulation tissue is present.

Acute Scrotal Pain

Acute scrotal pain is a medical emergency because it is necessary to rule out testicular torsion, which is a surgical emergency. The onset of testicular torsion is usually associated with acute, severe scrotal or testicular pain with nausea or vomiting. Detorsion is necessary within 4 to 6 hours to preserve testicular viability.

■ Etiology

The differential diagnosis of acute scrotal pain is shown in Box 11-3. Testicular torsion should be considered in any patient with acute-onset scrotal pain or swelling. Testicular torsion is usually divided into two subclasses: extravaginal torsion and intravaginal torsion. Extravaginal torsion is most common in neonates and is due to incomplete attachment of the testicular tunics to the scrotal wall, which allows the testis, epididymis, and tunica vaginalis to move freely within the scrotum. Intravaginal torsion is most common in

---

■ BOX 11-3 Differential Diagnosis of Acute Scrotal Pain

Testicular torsion
Epididymitis
Torsion of appendix testis or appendix epididymis
Incarcerated inguinal hernia
Testicular tumor
Idiopathic scrotal edema
Acute hydrocele
Henoch-Schönlein purpura
Spermatocele
Varicocele

adolescents, resulting from narrowing of the testicular mesentery from the cord onto the testis and epididymis. This abnormality leads to the **bell clapper deformity** and allows the testicle to twist within the tunica vaginalis.

Torsion of the appendix testis, in comparison to testicular torsion, is gradual in onset of pain and may be misinterpreted as epididymitis for this reason. The **blue-dot sign** is pathognomonic for torsion of the testicular appendages and is due to infarction in that region which can be seen through the scrotal wall.

■ Diagnosis

The basic workup for acute scrotal pain includes a history, physical examination with scrotal transillumination, urinalysis, and duplex Doppler ultrasonography.

Testicular torsion can be diagnosed from a history of acute-onset scrotal pain, swelling, negative cremasteric reflex with an abnormally elevated testicle, and relief of pain with successful manual detorsion during physical exam. A negative urinalysis result is often found, and decreased blood flow will be seen by color-flow Doppler ultrasonography. The bell clapper deformity may be present. Prehn's sign is often useful. In this test, manual elevation of the scrotum will result in a significant worsening of pain for patients with testicular torsion. This is referred to as a positive **Prehn's sign**. On the other hand, elevation of the acute scrotum in patients with acute epididymitis may produce an improvement in their pain. This is referred to as a negative Prehn's sign.

Torsion of the appendix testis or appendix epididymis can be differentiated from testicular torsion. In appendiceal torsion the onset of pain is gradual, and the patient generally has a positive cremasteric reflex. The blue-dot sign may be apparent, with decreased blood flow on color-flow Doppler ultrasonography. Urinalysis will be negative.

Conversely, epididymitis will show increased blood flow with color-flow Doppler ultrasonography, a positive Prehn's sign, a positive cremasteric reflex, and a positive urinalysis in prepubertal boys. In adolescents and young adults, epididymitis is related to sexual activity; therefore, the urinalysis is generally negative.

Henoch-Schönlein purpura is a small-vessel vasculitis that most commonly develops after an upper respiratory infection in children between the ages of 3 and 8. The IgA-dominant immune deposits can involve the vasculature of the testes or epididymis and cause scrotal pain.

An acute hydrocele is positive for transillumination, will have a positive cremasteric reflex, and is painless.

■ Treatment

The treatment for testicular torsion initially is manual detorsion. The direction of manual detorsion should be toward the thigh of the affected testis. For example, if the torsion is on the left side, detorsion should be counterclockwise. If this technique is successful, exploratory surgery is still necessary for fixation (orchiopexy) of the testes.

Torsion of the testicular appendages may be treated with non-steroidal anti-inflammatory drugs (NSAIDs), limited activity, and observation. If there is any question about the diagnosis, surgical exploration is warranted.

Epididymitis in this setting should be treated with NSAIDs, decreased activity, and prophylactic antibiotics (trimethoprim-sulfamethoxazole) until a voiding cystourethrogram (VCUG) can be performed. In prepubertal boys, a VCUG is warranted to rule out any bladder or kidney abnormalities when urinalysis is positive.

Paraphimosis

Paraphimosis is caused by chronic irritation of the foreskin. This irritation leads to tightening of the foreskin when it is pulled beyond the glans penis and remains stationary. This process leads to secondary pain because of swelling. Over time, arterial occlusion and necrosis of the glans penis can result.

■ Etiology and Diagnosis

The etiology of paraphimosis is usually iatrogenic, with retraction of the foreskin for urinary catheter placement without replacement of the foreskin to its natural position.

■ Treatment

Paraphimosis is treated initially with manual reduction. This reduction is done by applying pressure and an ice pack to the penis for 5 minutes, which helps decrease tissue swelling and the size of the glans penis. The foreskin is then manually pulled over the glans penis. This problem can be recurrent; thus, circumcision is advised after swelling has subsided. Antibiotics (such as a cephalosporin) should be taken during this waiting period.

If manual reduction is ineffective, a dorsal slit or circumcision under local anesthesia is necessary.

Microhematuria

Hematuria is defined as three or more red blood cells (RBC) per high-power field on microscopic examination of two of three

■ TABLE 11-1 Causes of Hematuria

Type	Cause
Glomerular hematuria	IgA nephropathy (Berger's disease)
	Mesangioproliferative glomerulonephritis
	Focal segmental proliferative glomerulonephritis
Nonglomerular hematuria	Exercise
	Bladder tumors
	Renal artery embolism/thrombosis
	Arteriovenous fistula
	Renal vein thrombosis
	Stones
	Urinary tract infections
	Renal cell carcinoma
	Papillary necrosis (consider in diabetics, blacks, and analgesic abusers)
	Injury
	Ureteral carcinoma
	Menstrual contamination
	Interstitial cystitis
	Extracorporeal shock-wave lithotripsy
Medications	Anticoagulants and analgesics

properly collected urine samples. Proper collection entails freshly voided, clean-catch, midstream urine samples. This microscopic evaluation should be used to confirm positive urine dipstick analysis of a patient with hematuria.

■ Etiology

The etiology of hematuria is complex and can be related to glomerular disease, nonglomerular disease, medications, familial diseases, exercise, and vascular disease. Table 11-1 presents the differential diagnosis of hematuria.

It is important to distinguish between nephritic and nephrotic syndrome when discussing glomerular disease. **Nephrotic syndrome** is defined by massive proteinuria (greater than 4 g/day), hypoalbuminemia (less than 3 g per 100 mL), generalized edema, hyperlipidemia, and hypercholesterolemia. This syndrome is usually caused by an increase in basement membrane permeability.

Nephritic syndrome is characterized by azotemia (increased blood urea nitrogen and creatinine levels), oliguria (decreased urine production), hypertension, and hematuria. This syndrome is an inflammatory process that causes glomerular capillary rupture.

IgA nephropathy (Berger's disease) is a nephritic syndrome that is the most common cause of glomerular hematuria. This disease is most commonly seen in children and young adult males following an upper respiratory infection, gastrointestinal infection, or exercise and usually self-resolves within 1 to 2 days.

Exercise can cause hematuria in those patients who are long-distance runners; such hematuria usually resolves quickly. The hematuria is usually of bladder or renal origin and may be the first underlying sign of glomerular disease; therefore, risk assessment may provide clues as to whether further testing is necessary.

Vascular disease is the primary cause for nonglomerular hematuria; therefore, it is necessary to rule out the four most common systemic diseases: diabetes mellitus, systemic lupus erythematosus (SLE), vasculitis, and amyloidosis. Renovascular and tubulointerstitial disorders may be other secondary causes of nonglomerular hematuria.

A family history of hematuria or bleeding easily may suggest a blood dyscrasia, whereas a history of urolithiasis or intermittent hematuria may suggest stone disease.

Anticoagulants used in excessive doses can cause hematuria, but not when maintained at therapeutic levels.

■ Diagnosis

The diagnosis of hematuria is based on two positive results of three freshly voided, midstream, clean-catch urine samples by dipstick examination. These positive dipsticks should be confirmed with microscopic examination of centrifuged urine, which should show three or more RBCs per high-power field. Patients diagnosed with hematuria should undergo a complete urologic evaluation, which includes a voided urine cytology, cystoscopy, imaging of the urinary tract via ultrasound, CT scan, or intravenous pyelogram (IVP), as well as a thorough history and physical exam.

It is important to question whether the hematuria is painful or painless, as well as which part of the stream is hematuric (beginning, end, or continuous).

Painful hematuria is more consistent with stone disease, cystitis, urinary tract infections (UTIs), or possible trauma; therefore, in addition to the exams discussed previously, a urinalysis is necessary. The patient may have a positive **Grey Turners sign** (flank discoloration) with renal trauma. Painless hematuria is always felt to be secondary to cancer of the urinary tract until proven otherwise. Painless hematuria may also be due to renal parenchymal disease (glomerular disease). The gold standard for diagnosis of IgA nephropathy (Berger's disease) is a renal biopsy, but a history of a recent upper respiratory infection or gastrointestinal infection will aid in that diagnosis. Renal cell carcinoma (RCC) accounts for 85% to 90% of renal cancers in adults and is more common in men in their sixth to seventh decades of life. It is important to note that the classic triad for RCC of costovertebral pain, palpable mass, and hematuria is only seen in 10% of patients.

Hematuria seen at the beginning of urination is commonly associated with anterior urethral bleeding. End-stream hematuria is associated with posterior urethral damage, bladder neck bleeding, or intravesical bleeding. Total hematuria is usually related to bleeding that occurs at the level of the bladder or above (i.e., ureter or kidney).

A good history will rule out other causes of red-colored urine, such as anthocyanin in beets and blackberries, chronic lead and mercury poisoning, rifampin, or phenothiazines. Brownish-black urine may be caused by use of laxatives (senna), Robaxin usage, methyldopa, or biochemical disorders such as alcaptonuria or tyrosinosis.

■ Treatment

IgA nephropathy (Berger's disease) is the most common cause of glomerular hematuria. This disease usually self-resolves after 2 to 4 days, but acute flare-ups may be treated with glucocorticoids. Twenty percent of these patients may progress to end-stage renal disease.

Nonglomerular hematuria is usually caused by primary urologic diseases, which commonly are tumors, stones, and UTIs. Seventy percent of UTIs are caused by *Escherichia coli*, yet other bacteria are also responsible. A good mnemonic for remembering the bacteria that cause UTIs is "SEEKS PP":

S = *Staphylococcus saprophyticus*
E = *Escherichia coli*
E = *Enterobacter*
K = *Klebsiella pneumoniae*
S = *Streptococcus faecalis*
P = *Proteus mirabilis*
P = *Pseudomonas aeruginosa*

The treatment of choice is either ciprofloxacin or levofloxacin. In pregnant women, fluoroquinolones should be avoided because they may cause damage to growing cartilage; sulfonamides should also be avoided because of increased risk of kernicterus if taken near the end of pregnancy. Ampicillin or gentamicin should be considered in these patients.

The treatment for urolithiasis depends on the size of the stone, as well as the location within the urinary tract. Stones that are less than 5 mm usually will pass without difficulty; therefore, hydration and analgesia are the mainstay of treatment. For stones less than 3 cm in diameter, extracorporeal shock-wave lithotripsy (ESWL), percutaneous nephrolithotomy (PCNL), or uretero-scopy may be warranted. The ureteral stones clinical guideline panel of the American Urologic Association (AUA) made recommendations for the treatment of stones depending on location: proximal, middle, or distal. Proximal stones are located in the ureteropelvic junction (UPJ), middle stones occur over the pelvic bone, and distal stones are located on the inferior border of the pelvic bone to the ureterovesical junction (UVJ).

For proximal stones smaller than 1 cm, the treatment of choice is ESWL or ureteroscopy. ESWL, ureteroscopy, or PCNL may be used for proximal stones larger than 1 cm, although ureteroscopy seems to be the procedure of choice. For middle stones smaller than 1 cm, the treatment of choice is either ESWL or uretero-scopy. Ureteroscopy is the procedure of choice for middle stones larger than 1 cm. Distal stones smaller than 1 cm may be treated effectively with either ureteroscopy or ESWL. Distal stones larg-er than 1 cm should be treated with ureteroscopy. Lastly, staghorn calculi are treated with PCNL.

The two most common renal tumors are renal cell carcinoma and Wilms' tumor (nephroblastoma). Renal cell carcinoma is the most common renal tumor in adults. The treatment of choice for RCC is a partial or radical nephrectomy. Because RCC is slow growing and has usually metastasized by diagnosis, it is necessary to rule out secondary sites of involvement. The most common secondary sites are the lungs (>50%), followed by bone (34%). For metastatic RCC, immunotherapy and radical nephrectomy are utilized.

Wilms' tumor is the most common primary renal tumor of childhood. It is generally unilateral and is diagnosed in children between 2 and 5 years old. Wilms' tumor is treated with both surgical removal of the affected kidney and chemotherapy. This dual treatment usually gives a 95% cure rate.

Urethral Catheterization

Urethral catheterization is performed to drain the bladder during and after surgical procedures, to assess urinary output, for urody-namic studies, for cystography, and to determine residual urine volume. The catheter can be left indwelling with a balloon to maintain position in the bladder. Alternatively, the bladder can be catheterized to drain a bladder and then the catheter removed.

In men, catheterization can be more challenging in the pres-ence of urethral stricture disease or in patients with prostate enlargement. In these patients, adequate lubrication injected into the urethra and a large-bore catheter (18F) should be used. Coudé-tipped (curved) catheters may be helpful to negotiate a high bladder neck, as seen in patients with benign prostate hyperplasia. It is important not to inflate the balloon prematurely in these cases because this can result in severe pain or urethral rupture. In these cases, one should wait until urine returns from the catheter to blow up the balloon.

In women, it may be difficult to identify the urethral meatus. The labia may need to be retracted. In some cases, a vaginal speculum may be required to locate the urethra. Similar to male catheterization, it is important not to blow up the catheter balloon prematurely. One should wait for urine return from the catheter before blowing up the balloon.

Another challenge is removal of the urinary catheter when the balloon will not deflate. First, the valve of the catheter should be inspected for problems. Second, one can cut the catheter proximal to the valve to evacuate the contents of the balloon. In cases where this is not successful, a guidewire can be passed down the balloon port in an attempt to puncture the balloon. Other options include placing a narrow cystoscope alongside the catheter to determine the source of the problem. In cases after radical prostatectomy, it may be possible to identify a suture wrapped around the catheter.

A Opportunities in Urology

Urology is a surgical specialty that encompasses the female urinary tract and the male reproductive organs. The discipline intertwines the disciplines of internal medicine, pediatrics, and gynecology. There are seven subspecialty areas of urology: pediatric urology, urologic oncology, infertility, renal transplantation, endourology, female urology, and neurourology. The discipline involves major and minor surgical procedures as well as office-based procedures.

Residency training in urology typically involves 5 or 6 years of clinical postgraduate education. The first year or two, depending on the program, is in general surgery. The remaining 36 to 48 months are spent in urology or other clinical disciplines relevant to urology. There are currently 122 approved residency programs and 8 military programs, which have their own matching process. There are approximately 230 entry-level positions offered through the American Urological Association (AUA) Matching Program. For more information about the match, applicants can contact the AUA:

Office of Education
American Urological Association
2425 West Loop South, Suite 333
Houston, Texas 77027-4207
(800) 282-7077
www.auanet.org

Additional information about the field of urology, as well as specific information about the process of certification by the American Board of Urology, can be obtained from the Board office:

The American Board of Urology
2216 Ivy Road, Suite 210
Charlottesville, VA 22903
(434) 979-0059
www.abu.org

The residency match occurs in January of the year prior to beginning urology residency training. This match occurs earlier than the typical March match of the National Resident Matching Program.

Because of this early match, applicants interview for programs between October and December. Programs and applicants submit match lists to the AUA, and the results are available by the end of January. Applicants who match in urology are typically required to complete their general surgery internship at the same institution. In most cases, this pre-urology year (or years) is arranged, and applicants are automatically matched in the respective surgery program. The results of the most recent match indicate a 70% match rate for graduates of U.S. medical schools. Match rates are significantly lower for students who have attended osteopathic or foreign medical schools.

HOW TO OBTAIN A UROLOGY RESIDENCY POSITION

As mentioned previously, urology is a very competitive program. Residency program directors are looking for applicants with strong board scores, class rank in the upper 25% of their class (preference given for Alpha Omega Alpha Honor Society election), strong letters of recommendation, and research experience in the field. Rotations in urology are also important, but, in general, most urology programs think that 2 months of urology electives is the maximum amount needed to be performed by students. These audition electives are important and can be used by applicants to further their commitment to the field as well as obtain a letter of support from the department chairperson or program director.

Preparation of the application materials is also important. Applicants should pay particular attention to their curriculum vitae (CV) and personal statement. The CV should be an honest assessment of the applicant's experiences to date, including research undertaken and honors received. The personal statement should be a one-page concise statement of the applicant's motivation for entering the field of urology. The statement should be free from spelling and grammatical errors because this would reflect a careless applicant.

The residency interview is an important part of the application process. Typically, the applicant will have 5 to 10 short interviews (20 to 30 minutes each) with faculty members or residents or both. Interviewers are looking for applicants with sincere interest in urology, humanism, and cooperation with the staff and residents. On the other hand, the interview provides the applicant with a chance to preview the residency program and have his or her questions answered. For instance, Is the quality of the program and clinical material adequate? Are the residents exposed to all aspects of urology? Is there a structured, didactic teaching program with conferences, journal clubs, case presentations, conferences, and other educational activities? Based on these questions, the applicant can make an informed decision about the merits of each program.

B Questions and Answers in Urology

QUESTIONS

The following questions were constructed to reflect the current content and format of licensure examinations taken by medical students. These questions are also likely to be useful for interns preparing to take in-service and licensure examinations.

1. A 47-year-old gravida 4 para 4 woman complains of urinary incontinence. She has urinary urgency and nocturia three times per week. Urine loss is described as moderate, lasting for several seconds, and is often associated with change in position. She adds that incontinence can be precipitated by running water, such as in the kitchen while washing dishes. She notes no incontinence related to coughing or laughing. She has a palpable thyroid gland without masses. Cardiac examination reveals a midsystolic click, while pulmonary auscultation reveals no evidence of rales or wheezes. Gastrointestinal examination reveals tenderness to deep palpation in the most inferior portions of the right and left lower quadrants without evidence of guarding or rebound tenderness. Bowel sounds are normoactive. Rectal examination is guaiac negative with stool in the vault. Pelvic examination reveals no evidence of structural abnormalities. Which of the following is the most likely diagnosis?

   A. Cystocele
   B. Overflow incontinence
   C. Stress incontinence
   D. Urge incontinence
   E. Urethrocele

2. A 74-year-old man with a history of diabetes mellitus and hypothyroidism presents for evaluation of intermittent gross hematuria with small clots noted upon urination. He complains of nocturia three times per night and decreased force of urinary stream with hesitancy. He is a nonsmoker, but admits to one beer per week for the past 20 years. His medications include an oral hypoglycemic agent and a synthetic thyroid hormone preparation. Physical examination reveals no evidence of rubs, murmurs, or gallops. Pulmonary auscultation reveals decreased breath sounds at the bases bilaterally. Gastrointestinal examination reveals some tenderness along the sigmoid colon without evidence of guarding or rebound tenderness. Rectal examination is guaiac positive with stool in the vault. A small internal hemorrhoid is noted in the left lateral position.

Urine analysis reveals 2+ hematuria with no evidence of leukocytes or nitrates. Kidney and bladder sonography reveal no evidence of hydronephrosis. The bladder is smooth. Which of the following is the most likely diagnosis?

A. Acute prostatitis
B. Bladder carcinoma
C. Prostate hyperplasia
D. Renal calculi
E. Urinary tract infection

3. A 91-year-old man who is wheelchair-bound and in a nursing home has a urinary catheter placed because of a prolonged history of enuresis and daytime urinary incontinence. His current medical problems include diabetes mellitus, hypertension, and congestive heart failure, and he has a history of myocardial infarction 2 years ago. His current medications include glyburide, atenolol, and Lasix. On a recent urine culture in the nursing home, the patient is noted to have 75,000 colony-forming units/mL of *Escherichia coli*. In which of the following scenarios should the patient receive antibiotic therapy?

A. After removal of the urinary catheter
B. Gross hematuria develops
C. Pyuria develops
D. The patient develops fever and chills
E. Urine culture reveals a second organism

4. A 27-year-old man and his 24-year-old wife present for a wellness examination. Both individuals are healthy and without medical problems. The male partner notes that he was able to father a child 2 years ago with a former girlfriend. Physical examination of the male partner reveals an uncircumcised phallus with a patent meatus. Both testicles are descended without evidence of mass lesions. Cremaster reflex is noted on the left side but is absent on the right. The female partner was examined by her gynecologist, who noted that there were no structural abnormalities. Which of the following is the optimal timing of intercourse to achieve conception for this couple?

A. Once weekly
B. Twice weekly during the midmenstrual cycle
C. Twice daily during the midmenstrual cycle
D. Three times on the day of ovulation

5. A 3-year-old boy presents for evaluation of an abdominal mass found by his parents during his nighttime bath. The parents note that the child has recently had some bouts of vomiting and intermittent right-sided abdominal pain. The patient appears well. Physical examination reveals no evidence or rales, rhonchi, or wheezing. Cardiac examination reveals no murmurs or gallops. Gastrointestinal evaluation notes a right-sided abdominal mass that does not cross the midline. Urine analysis shows no evidence of

hematuria, nitrites, or leukocytes. Which of the following is the most appropriate next step in the evaluation of this patient?

A. Barium enema
B. Cystoscopy
C. Retrograde urethrogram
D. Transabdominal sonography
E. Ureteroscopic evaluation and biopsy

6. A 24-year-old woman complains of vaginal growths on her labia for the past 4 months. These growths have persisted and are not painful. She had a similar occurrence of such lesions at age 18, which responded to medical therapy. She is sexually active with multiple male partners and intermittently uses condoms as contraception. Pelvic examination reveals several papules with raised margins and irregular borders. The lesions involve the labia bilaterally. Rectal examination reveals no evidence of hemorrhoids. Which of the following is the most likely diagnosis?

A. Chancroid
B. Condyloma acuminata
C. Condyloma lata
D. Genital herpes
E. Molluscum contagiosum

7. A 31-year-old man with a history of depression has recently begun a sexual relationship with a new female partner. Since the beginning of this relationship, he has had a pattern of ejaculation that occurs with minimal sexual stimulation, often immediately with vaginal penetration. Physical examination reveals an uncircumcised penis with a patent urethral meatus. The testicles are descended bilaterally without evidence of palpable masses. Cremasteric reflexes are present bilaterally. Which of the following is the most appropriate treatment for this condition?

A. Behavioral techniques
B. Directive marital therapy
C. Pharmacologic therapy
D. Psychodynamic approaches
E. Surgical resection

8. A 41-year-old man complains of a 4-day history of right scrotal pain. He is sexually active with multiple partners and admits to recent unprotected sexual encounters. He has a history of non-insulin-dependent diabetes mellitus, takes an oral medication, and maintains good sugar control. Cardiac examination reveals a regular rate and rhythm. There is no evidence of rubs, murmurs, or gallops. Pulmonary auscultation reveals good breath sounds bilaterally. Gastrointestinal evaluation reveals normoactive bowel sounds. Bilateral cremasteric reflexes are intact. The right scrotum is erythematous and edematous. The testis is palpable without masses, but is tender to the touch, as is the epididymis. The left scrotum is without

tenderness, edema, or erythema. The left testis is without masses. Urinalysis reveals nitrites and leukocytes with trace hematuria. Which of the following is the most likely etiology of this condition?

A. Antegrade spread from the bladder
B. Hematogenous
C. Lymphatic
D. Retrograde reflux from the prostate and seminal vesicle
E. Urinary incontinence

9. A 63-year-old man who has a 60 pack-year history of smoking complains of gross hematuria. Physical examination of the heart, lungs, and abdomen is within normal limits. The prostate is approximately 40 grams and is symmetric. Intravenous pyelography reveals normal kidneys and ureters bilaterally. A small filling defect is noted within the floor of the urinary bladder. Cystoscopy is performed and reveals a sessile, papillary growth approximately 2 cm by 4 cm proximal to the left ureteral orifice. Biopsies of the lesion are taken and are most likely to reveal:

A. Adenocarcinoma
B. Carcinoid tumor
C. Sarcoma
D. Squamous cell carcinoma
E. Transitional cell carcinoma

10. A 27-year-old man complains of a painless lump in his right groin. He has a prior surgical history of right orchiopexy at age 4. He has no other medical conditions and takes no medications. Cardiac examination reveals a regular rate and rhythm. Pulmonary auscultation reveals no rales, rhonchi, or wheezing. Gastrointestinal examination reveals normoactive bowel sounds. The right testis has a 1.5-cm area of induration on the posterior surface. The right epididymis and vas deferens are palpable. The left testis has no areas of induration. The left epididymis and vas deferens are palpable. Ultrasound of the right testicle reveals a well-circumscribed hypoechoic area within the right testicle. Chest x-ray reveals no evidence of effusions, masses, or infiltrates. Which of the following is the most likely diagnosis?

A. Embryonal carcinoma
B. Endodermal sinus tumor
C. Seminoma
D. Teratoma
E. Teratocarcinoma

11. A 33-year-old man presents to his physician for evaluation of right scrotal pain. He has no prior medical or surgical history. Physical examination reveals a 2-cm solid mass in the lower pole of the right testicle. Transillumination of the right hemiscrotum is also noted.

Which of the following is the most appropriate initial step in the management of this condition?

A. Chemotherapy
B. Inguinal orchiectomy
C. Radiotherapy
D. Radiotherapy and chemotherapy
E. Transscrotal orchiectomy

12. A 66-year-old man with biopsy-proven adenocarcinoma of the prostate has opted for treatment with an LH-RH agonist and an antiandrogen agent. He still suffers from significant bone pain. Which of the following agents might provide him with relief of bone pain?

A. Estramustine phosphate
B. Growth factors
C. Paclitaxel
D. Retinoids
E. Strontium-89 chloride

13. A 66-year-old man with an elevated prostate-specific antigen level undergoes a prostate needle biopsy. Pathology reveals a Gleason 3+4 adenocarcinoma on all slides. He desires not to undergo surgical or medical treatment for his disease. He fully understands the risks and benefits of his decision. Regarding the relative propensity for bony metastasis from prostate cancer, which of the following is the site with the highest frequency of metastasis from this disease?

A. Femur
B. Humerus
C. Pelvis and sacrum
D. Ribs
E. Scapula

14. Investigators are trying to determine the usefulness of a new assay based on the enzyme telomerase to determine the presence of superficial bladder cancer. This assay is based on the presence of telomerase in voided urine specimens. Patients who have indwelling urinary catheters were excluded from the present study. The following data from 200 patients are obtained:

Telomerase	Cancer Present	Cancer Absent
Positive	60	40
Negative	20	80

In this study, the specificity is

A. 10%
B. 20%
C. 50%
D. 67%
E. 96%

15. A 28-year-old man has been your patient for 3 years. During that period of time, he has been treated for an upper respiratory tract infection and sinusitis. He presents to your office complaining of curvature of his penis, with erection and penile pain for the last 24 hours. The patient stated that he had intercourse about 26 hours ago, then developed penile curvature with the following erection and penile pain. He notes that there is a small palpable lump along the penile shaft. Detailed information regarding which of the following entities would be helpful in the workup and management of this patient?

A. History of arthritis
B. History of epididymitis
C. Recent use of alpha-blocking agents
D. Recent use of beta-agonist agents
E. Recent use of a vacuum-constricting erection device

16. Further questioning of a 42-year-old patient with Peyronie's disease reveals no recent use of intracavernosal injections and no underlying immunologic disorder. Physical examination reveals a dense fibrous plaque near the dorsal midline of the shaft. Which of the following is the most likely anatomic location of this plaque?

A. Corpus cavernosum
B. Penile urethra
C. Prostatic urethra
D. Tunica albuginea overlying the corpus cavernosum
E. Tunica vaginalis

Questions 17 and 18 refer to the following case presentation:

A 50-year-old man who you have been seeing in your office for 5 years returns with a new onset of left flank pain radiating to the left groin. He has a history of gout and is taking allopurinol. He is afebrile. His physical exam reveals a normal abdominal exam, but he does have left costovertebral tenderness. His creatinine level is 1.1 mg/dL.

17. Which of the following exams would be the *least* likely to demonstrate a renal stone (urolithiasis) in this patient?

A. Computed tomography of the abdomen and pelvis
B. Helical (spiral) computed tomographic scan of the abdomen and pelvis
C. Intravenous pyelogram
D. Radiograph of the abdomen (KUB)
E. Ultrasound of the kidneys and bladder

18. Which of the following is most likely found on urine dipstick and/or urinalysis?

A. Coffin-lid crystals
B. Hexagonal crystals
C. Microhematuria
D. Square crystals with a notched corner
E. Urine pH = 6.8

19. A 29-year-old man falls from a second-story window. He is found unconscious by emergency medical services. He is brought to the emergency department for treatment. The patient is unable to provide a urine specimen. Which of the following would be an absolute contraindication to placement of a Foley catheter prior to further evaluation?

    A. History of transurethral resection of the prostate (TURP)
    B. Occult blood found on rectal exam
    C. Scrotal hematoma
    D. Severe abdominal pain
    E. Severe back pain

20. A 57-year-old African American man comes to clinic for an annual physical examination. He has no complaints. Digital rectal examination reveals a 1.5-cm rock-hard discrete nodule. What is the next appropriate step in the management of this patient?

    A. Measurement of prostate-specific antigen (PSA)
    B. Transrectal needle biopsy
    C. Begin a course of flutamide
    D. Prostatectomy
    E. Begin a course of nilutamide

21. A 47-year-old Asian man complains of a 1-month history of not being able to function sexually with his wife, and his marriage is suffering as a result. His past medical history is significant for hypertension and bipolar disorder. He also admits to having a 30 pack-year history of smoking. He also admits that his wife has recently cheated on him with a 26-year-old man. He complains of having difficulty obtaining an erection, achieving an orgasm, and ejaculating. Laboratory tests results are as follows:

    Testosterone = 375 mg/dL
    Glucose = 111 mg/dL
    Cholesterol = 218 mg/dL
    T3 = 0.4 ng/dL
    T4 = 8 µg/dL
    Triglycerides = 100 mg/dL
    Prostate-specific antigen = 2 ng/mL
    Duplex ultrasound showed no arterial narrowing.
    Nocturnal penile tumescence (NPT) test showed positive erection during REM sleep.

The most appropriate treatment is which of the following?

    A. Counseling
    B. Sildenafil citrate
    C. Vacuum erection device
    D. Hormone replacement therapy
    E. Injection therapy with papaverine

22. A 55-year-old man undergoes prostate needle biopsy for a PSA of 4.2 ng/mL. He has no prior medical or surgical history. BMI is the 50th percentile for age. AUA symptom score is 6. SHIM score is 21. Physical examination of the heart, lungs, and abdomen are unremarkable. Prostate is 30 grams and without nodules. Pathology reveals a Gleason 3+3=6 prostate cancer in 2 of 12 cores. What is the most appropriate intervention for this patient?

    A. Radical prostatectomy
    B. External beam radiotherapy
    C. Transperineal brachytherapy with palladium seeds
    D. 1-month course of fluoroquinolone antibiotic
    E. 1-month course of fluoroquinolone antibiotic and NSAID

23. Two patients, a man and a woman, present to your office after they met on the Androgen Awareness Chatroom website. The woman is concerned because she has facial hair and frontal balding, and the man is concerned because he has gynoid fat distribution and a high-pitched voice. What is a single etiology that would account for both their presentations?

    A. 21-alpha hydroxylase deficiency
    B. 11-beta hydroxylase deficiency
    C. 3-beta hydroxysteroid dehydrogenase
    D. 17-alpha hydroxylase deficiency
    E. Anabolic steroid use

24. A 16-year-old boy presents to the emergency department with severe acute onset of right testicular pain that began 2 hours ago. There was no history of trauma to the testicle, and the patient reports being in good health with no recent illness. Upon examination, the patient was afebrile, and the right testicle was swollen, painful, and high riding with a horizontal lie. Elevation of the testicle by the examiner provided some relief of pain. What is the most likely diagnosis?

    A. Acute epididymitis
    B. Acute bacterial prostatitis
    C. Henoch-Schönlein purpura
    D. Testicular carcinoma
    E. Testicular torsion

25. Prostate-specific antigen is

    A. A protease inhibitor
    B. A serine protease
    C. Complexed to trypsin
    D. Expressed by smooth muscle cells
    E. Expressed by striated muscle cells

ANSWER KEY

1. **D**	10. **C**	19. **C**
2. **C**	11. **B**	20. **B**
3. **D**	12. **E**	21. **A**
4. **B**	13. **C**	22. **A**
5. **D**	14. **D**	23. **C**
6. **D**	15. **E**	24. **E**
7. **A**	16. **D**	25. **B**
8. **D**	17. **D**	
9. **E**	18. **C**	

ANSWERS

1. **D. This patient has urge incontinence. This condition is associated with urinary urgency and nocturia. Patients typically complain of losing large amounts of urine associated with changes in position and when near running water (in this case, while washing the dishes). The etiology of this condition is loss of bladder inhibition. No structural abnormalities are associated with this type of incontinence.** Cystocele is an outpouching of the bladder due to loss of pelvic support or prolapse of the urethra. This condition is associated with urine loss during increases in intra-abdominal pressure, especially with coughing and sneezing. The cystocele is often noted upon rectovaginal examination. Overflow incontinence is associated with neurologic conditions such as Parkinson's disease and cerebrovascular accidents. Patients complain of dribbling small amounts of urine associated with increases in abdominal pressure. Stress incontinence is associated with small amounts of urine loss associated with coughing, laughing, sneezing, or physical activity and can occur in any position (upright or supine). Urethrocele is descent of the urethra due to detachment or prolapse. This condition is often noted on rectovaginal examination and is associated with urine loss of small volumes during periods of increased intra-abdominal pressure (coughing, sneezing, or straining to move bowels).

2. **C. In this patient of greater than 70 years of age, there is a 70% chance that he has benign prostatic hyperplasia. In addition to urinary obstructive symptoms, such as nocturia, frequency, urgency, and decreased force of stream, intermittent gross hematuria is also possible.** Acute prostatitis can be associated with intermittent gross hematuria, but is more frequently associated with

fever, low back pain, and a tender prostate upon digital rectal examination. Bladder carcinoma can be associated with either gross or microscopic hematuria, as well as irritative or obstructive urinary symptoms. This patient has a normal kidney and bladder sonogram and is a nonsmoker, which places him at low risk for this disease. Renal calculi are usually associated with hydronephrosis or hydroureter, as well as the presence of a stone on sonography. Microhematuria is more commonly seen with this condition. Urinary tract infection is unlikely, given the urinalysis findings of negative nitrates and leukocytes.

3. **D. All patients with an indwelling catheter will eventually develop bacteriuria. After the catheter has been in place for approximately 10 days, nearly all patients will have asymptomatic bacteriuria. This patient should not receive antibiotic therapy unless he becomes symptomatic and develops fever or chills. Treatment of patients with bacteriuria without symptoms will lead to development of resistant organisms, which will ultimately become a problem when the patient develops a true urinary tract infection.** This patient should not receive antibiotic therapy when the catheter is removed unless there is clinical evidence of infection. Gross hematuria in the absence of a positive urinalysis or urine culture should not be treated with antibiotics. As mentioned previously, pyuria in the absence of clinical evidence of infection should not be treated with antibiotics. Patients with indwelling Foley catheters who receive a urine culture may grow two organisms. These individuals should not receive antibiotic therapy unless they have clinical evidence of infection.

4. **B. After ovulation, the ovum remains viable for approximately 48 hours. It is during this time that fertilization should take place. The optimal timing for intercourse should be twice weekly during the middle of the menstrual cycle. Sperm remain viable for approximately 40 to 72 hours after intercourse.** Intercourse once weekly might allow for a miss of the 48-hour window of ovum viability for fertility. Intercourse twice daily during the midmenstrual cycle may produce smaller amounts of viable semen and limit chances of conception. Intercourse three times during the day of ovulation may produce smaller amounts of viable semen and limit chances of conception. It is often difficult for a woman to carefully calculate her exact day of ovulation, which will further limit this particular strategy.

5. **D. Wilm's' tumor is the most common kidney tumor in children and can be associated with genitourinary anomalies, hemihypertrophy, and sporadic aniridia. Patients are usually 2 to 5 years old at diagnosis and present with a unilateral abdominal mass. Associated symptoms can include nausea and vomiting. Ultrasound can show an intra-renal mass, while CT scanning can reveal a heterogenous mass arising from the kidney.** The differential

diagnosis of this condition does not include gastrointestinal causes. Therefore, barium enema is not a useful study. Bladder tumors or lesions are not likely in this age group. Therefore, cystoscopy is not indicated. A retrograde urethrogram is indicated in patients with significant voiding symptoms to evaluate the contour of the urethra. Ureteral pathology is rare in children. Thus, retrograde ureteroscopy is not indicated in this patient.

6. **D. Genital herpes is associated with a variable number of papules with raised margins and an irregular border. There is no associated lymphadenopathy or induration. Treatment involves topical and/or oral antiviral agents.** Chancroid is associated with papules or pustules that are red and irregularly shaped on a yellow or grey base. The regional lymph nodes are often tender. Condyloma acuminata (venereal warts) are soft, fleshy growths on the vulva, cervix, perineum, and/or anus. The lesions can be single or multiple. Diagnosis is made on physical examination and confirmed with biopsy of the lesions. Treatment of uncomplicated warts can be accomplished with topical podophyllin. Treatment with 5-fluorouracil, cryosurgery, or surgical excision is required for more extensive lesions. Condyloma lata are found in syphilis and are flat lesions that are red and firm. They have a broad base and are nontender. Molluscum contagiosum is associated with lesions that have central umbilication and are more common over the lower abdomen. The appearance of these lesions is described as yellow and cheesy.

7. **A. It is estimated that 30% of the male population suffers from premature ejaculation. This condition is more prevalent in the young and those with a new sexual partner. This dysfunction is most amenable to cure when behavioral techniques are used in the treatment protocol.** Directive marital therapy is effective in the treatment of dyspareunia. Pharmacologic therapy is not considered to be a primary treatment of premature ejaculation. Psychodynamic approaches are considered to be effective therapy for dyspareunia. Surgical resection is not considered to be an effective therapy for premature ejaculation.

8. **D. This individual has acute nonspecific epididymitis, which is probably secondary to infection that has its origin in the prostate and seminal vesicles and then spreads in a retrograde manner to the epididymis.** Antegrade passage of bacteria is not a common pathogenesis for acute epididymitis. Acute epididymitis rarely results from hematogenous spread. Acute epididymitis rarely results from lymphatic spread. Urinary incontinence is not part of the pathogenesis of acute epididymitis.

9. **E. The incidence of bladder cancer in the United States is approximately 60,000 cases per year, with a median age of onset of 65 years. Smoking accounts for 50% of the risk. Greater than 90%**

of tumors are derived from transitional epithelium. Hematuria is the initial sign in approximately 90% of patients. Superficial tumors can be removed at cystoscopy. Adenocarcinoma represents 2% of all bladder carcinomas. Carcinoid tumors represent less than 1% of all bladder carcinomas. Sarcoma represents less than 1% of all bladder carcinomas. Squamous cell carcinoma represents approximately 3% of all bladder cancers.

10. C. This patient probably has testicular carcinoma. The peak incidence is between the ages of 20 and 40 years. Cryptorchid testis testes are at increased risk. Early orchiopexy does not protect against development of testicular cancer. Seminoma accounts for 50% of cases and is the most common pathology seen. Ultrasound often reveals a well-circumscribed hypoechoic area within the testicle. Embryonal cell carcinoma (20% of cases) is a nonseminomatous germ cell tumor of the testis. Endodermal sinus tumor (5%) is a common testis tumor in newborn males. Teratoma (15%) is a nonseminomatous germ cell tumor of the testis. Teratocarcinoma (20%) is a nonseminomatous germ cell tumor of the testis.

11. B. For all stages of seminoma, treatment first involves inguinal orchiectomy for histopathologic diagnosis and staging. For higher-stage disease, retroperitoneal lymph node dissection is undertaken. When positive lymph nodes are found, radiotherapy and chemotherapy are instituted. Chemotherapy is not the primary therapy for seminoma. Radiotherapy is not the primary therapy for seminoma. Chemotherapy and radiotherapy may be required for the treatment of advanced seminoma following orchiectomy. Transscrotal orchiectomy is not indicated in the treatment of testicular cancer. It is possible that during removal of the tumor by this approach lymphatic seeding of tumor cells could occur.

12. E. Strontium-89 chloride is a radiopharmaceutical agent similar to calcium and can provide palliative relief of pain from bony metastasis through calcium metabolic pathways. Approximately 75% of patients experience some pain relief, and 20% are rendered pain free. Estramustine is a nitrogen mustard that binds to microtubules and may have promise in the treatment of metastatic prostate cancer. Growth factors such as inhibitors of epidermal growth factors may show promise in the treatment of metastatic prostate cancer. Paclitaxel binds to cytoplasmic microtubules and inhibits the invasiveness of prostate cancer cells in vitro. Retinoids bind to nuclear receptors and promote cellular differentiation and may show promise in the treatment of metastatic prostate cancer.

13. C. When prostate cancer metastasizes beyond the organ of origin, the primary tumor initially spreads to bone, with the axial skeleton being the most frequent site of involvement. Sites of metastasis in order of frequency are the pelvis and sacrum, spine,

and femur. The femur is the third most common site of metastasis from prostate cancer. The humerus is an uncommon site of metastasis from prostate cancer. The ribs are the fourth most common site of metastasis from prostate cancer. The scapula is the fifth most common site of metastasis from prostate cancer.

14. **D. Specificity is the true negative rate. Specificity is defined as the probability of a negative test when the disease is absent. For the present study, this can be determined by the following formula: Specificity = (True Negatives/True Negatives) + False Positives. In this case, specificity is (80/80) + 40 = 67%. Sensitivity, on the other hand, is defined as positivity in disease and can also be determined by the following formula: Sensitivity = (True Positives/True Positives) + False Negatives.**

15. **E. A detailed history should be obtained from the patient presenting with penile pain and curvature on erection, which may suggest Peyronie's disease. Physicians should elicit information regarding recent penile trauma, medication use (especially beta-blocking agents), intracavernosal injections, use of a vacuum constriction device, and presence of underlying diseases, such as scleroderma.** A history of scleroderma may be noted in this patient. Epididymitis is not associated with Peyronie's disease. Recent use of alpha-agonist agents may be associated with this disorder. Beta-blocking agents can cause erectile dysfunction, which may lead to Peyronie's disease.

16. **D. The physical findings of a palpable penile plaque near the dorsal midline of the penile shaft in combination with the patient's complaint of penile curvature and penile pain suggest Peyronie's disease as the likely diagnosis. This condition is related to inflammation of the tunica albuginea overlying the corpus cavernosum, resulting in fibrosis and plaque formation.** Plaques are not located in the corpus cavernosum. Plaques are not located in the penile urethra. Plaques are not located in the prostatic urethra. Plaques are not located in the tunica vaginalis.

17. **D. Renal stones caused by uric acid are nonopaque or radiolucent. These stones are not visible on plain x-ray. Radiolucent stones make up 20% of all cases of urolithiasis.** CT scan will show most uric acid stones if they are large enough to be visualized on the slices. CT scan will also show the presence of hydronephrosis. Helical CT scans, in addition to the techniques available to regular CT scans, can visualize smaller renal stones. Intravenous pyelogram will show a radiolucent filling defect, demonstrating a stone. Ultrasound examination of renal stones show a density with a trailing shadow.

18. **C. With most cases of urolithiasis, some degree of microhematuria exists due to inflammation of the mucosa. Even though stone disease is presumed, one should exclude other causes of**

microhematuria, which include infection and neoplasia. Although it is possible to have triple phosphate crystals present (a sign of chronic infection), given the history of gout, uric acid crystals are much more probable. Hexagonal crystals are seen with cystinuria. This is a very rare disease, and these crystals would not be found in someone who does not exhibit other signs of cystinuria. Square crystals with a notched corner, which look like the state of Utah, are cholesterol crystals. These crystals are very rare. Uric acid crystals precipitate at a pH less than 5.5. In a patient who is experiencing uric acid stones, one would expect the pH to be lower than 5.5.

19. **C. Scrotal hematoma, blood at the urethral meatus, or high-riding prostate on digital rectal examination are all absolute contraindications to the placement of a catheter without evaluating the urethra because these are all signs of urethral disruption. A retrograde urethrogram should be performed.** A patient who had a transurethral resection of the prostate (TURP) may have had a recurrence of his prostatic hypertrophy and the stressful situation put him into urinary retention. The urethra is still present in patients who had a TURP, and a Foley catheter can be placed. Occult blood is often not found on rectal exam of trauma patients because a complete rectal exam is often not performed (i.e., not looking for hemorrhoids). If a high-riding prostate is found, a Foley catheter should not be placed; however, occult blood in the stool is not a contraindication. Abdominal pain in itself is not a contraindication to Foley placement because the patient may be complaining from urinary retention. It is important to evaluate these patients for the presence of hematuria to exclude bladder perforation or renal injury. Back pain does not indicate a urethral disruption. However, if additional signs of scrotal or flank hematoma are present, one may consider a retrograde urethrogram to exclude retroperitoneal tracking of urine or blood.

20. **B. The incidence of prostatic cancer increases with age, and this type of cancer has been found to be most common in African American males. Adenocarcinoma of the prostate typically arises at the periphery of the gland; therefore, digital rectal examination is one of the best screening tests for prostate cancer. Upon palpation of a mass, transrectal needle biopsy should be used to confirm the diagnosis. Spread of prostate cancer is by local extension, with the most common location of metastasis being the axial skeleton. Widespread bone metastases may respond to several therapies, including androgen ablation, orchiectomy, LHRH agonists, or antiandrogens such as flutamide.** This patient should have a prostate needle biopsy based on the finding of an abnormal digital rectal examination. Flutamide is an antiandrogen used to treat advanced prostate cancer. Prostatectomy is the gold-standard treatment for organ-confined prostate cancer. Nilutamide is an antiandrogen used to treat advanced prostate cancer.

21. **A.** Although the patient has multiple risk factors for a physiological cause for his impotence, the lab values are all within normal limits and the NPT showed that he *is* able to obtain an erection. Because his NPT was normal, there is a high likelihood of emotional and psychological causes for the impotence. Sildenafil is used in those patients with true erectile dysfunction as a result of a physiologic abnormality. A vacuum erection device is useful in patients with vasculogenic erectile dysfunction. Hormone replacement is not likely to benefit the patient with psychogenic impotence. Intracavernosal injection therapy is appropriate for patients with vasculogenic or neurogenic impotence.

22. **A.** This patient is relatively young and healthy. He appears to have localized prostate cancer on the basis of his prostate needle biopsy. His PSA is less than 10 ng/mL and he has no palpable disease on digital rectal examination. He is an excellent candidate for a radical prostatectomy because his life expectancy is greater than 10 years. External beam radiotherapy is not considered a first-line treatment for a young, healthy man with apparent organ-confined prostate cancer. Transperineal brachytherapy is currently evolving into a first-line treatment for localized prostate cancer; however, the treatment of choice for this patient still remains radical prostatectomy. This patient has prostate cancer by virtue of the findings at prostate needle biopsy. He should be treated definitively for this condition. This patient does not demonstrate the finding of inflammatory cells on biopsy to suggest the diagnosis of chronic prostatitis.

23. **C.** 3-beta hydroxylase deficiency results in an inability to convert pregnenolone to progesterone and an inability to convert dehydroepiandrosterone (DHEA) further down the androgen synthesis pathway. The result is an accumulation of DHEA and its sulfate, DHEAS. Both of these have a mild androgenic quality that results in "too much androgen in females and not enough androgen in males," resulting in the patients in this question. Patients with 21-alpha hydroxylase deficiency do not make 17 hydroxyprogesterone and present with salt wasting and adrenal insufficiency at the time of birth. The pathway is shifted then to make more androgens than normal. Female infants present with ambiguous genitalia from excess androgens. Patients with 11-beta hydroxylase deficiency present with similar symptoms of androgen excess because precursors are shunted toward androgen production. Patients with 17-alpha hydroxylase deficiency would not be able to make androgens. Patients with anabolic steroid use would both present with masculinization, though the man may present with gynecomastia and shrunken testicles once he stops their use.

24. **E.** Testicular torsion is the correct answer in this scenario and is indeed a urologic emergency. A high-riding testicle in a horizontal lie for which elevation of the testicle provides relief is the classic presentation of testicular torsion. The critical time of ischemia

for testicular torsion is 4 hours, and if a gangrenous testicle is missed, the patient will be at high risk for sterility due to his body mounting an autoimmune response to his own sperm. Appropriate management is immediate bilateral orchiopexy because the contralateral testicle is also at an increased risk of torsion. Epididymitis is unlikely in this scenario due to the lack of fever or systemic illness in this patient. Epididymitis is not a urologic emergency and can be treated with oral antibiotics. Prostatitis is unlikely given the clinical presentation and the lack of urinary symptoms. Henoch-Schönlein purpura is associated with a purpuric rash on the scrotum and fever. Testicular cancer is most commonly found in young men, but the usual presentation is a painless testicular mass.

25. **B. Prostate-specific antigen (PSA) is a serine protease that liquefies the seminal coagulum by degrading proteins in the semen.** Protease inhibitors are used to treat patients with HIV disease. PSA is complexed to α_1-antichymotrypsin. PSA is expressed in small amounts by cells of cloacal origin. PSA is not expressed by striated muscle cells.

C Commonly Prescribed Medications in Urology

ADULT DOSES OF COMMONLY USED MEDICATIONS

Acetohydroxamic acid 250 mg PO TID or QID (for struvite stones)

Allopurinol 300 mg PO q day (for uric acid lithiasis)

Aminobenzoate potassium (Potaba) 3 g PO q 6 hours or 2 g PO q 4 hours for at least 2 to 3 months (for Peyronie's disease)

Bicalutamide (Casodex) 50 mg PO q day (for combined androgen deprivation for prostate cancer)

Bicitra (sodium citrate) 10–30 mEq PO BID to QID (each mL of solution yields 1 mEq sodium and 1 mEq bicarbonate)

Cellulose sodium phosphate 5 g PO BID or TID (for type I absorptive hypercalciuria)

Chlorpromazine 25 mg PO TID (for hyperchloremic metabolic acidosis associated with urinary diversion or augmentation)

Cholestyramine 400 mg PO TID or 300 mg PO QID (for enteric hyperoxaluria)

Colchicine 0.6 mg PO TID or 1.2 mg PO BID after meals (for Peyronie's disease)

D-Penicillamine 250–1000 mg PO QID (for cystinuria) and give with pyridoxine 25–50 mg PO q day

Doxazosin (Cardura) 1–8 mg PO QD (for BPH)

Dutasteride (Avodart) 0.5 mg PO q day (for BPH)

Finasteride (Proscar) 5 mg PO q day (for BPH)

5-Fluorouracil (5%) topically BID for 3 to 4 weeks (for CIS of penis)

Flutamide (Eulexin) 250 mg PO TID (for combined androgen deprivation for prostate cancer)

Goserelin acetate (Zoladex) 3.6 mg SQ q month or 10.8 mg SQ every 3 months (for prostate cancer)

Hydrochlorothiazide 50 mg PO BID (for renal leak hypercalciuria or type I absorptive hypercalciuria)

Ketoconazole (Nizoral) 200–400 mg PO TID (for androgen deprivation for prostate cancer)

Leuprolide acetate (Lupron) 7.5 mg IM q month or 22.5 mg IM q 3 months or 30 mg IM q 4 months (for prostate cancer)

Magnesium gluconate 250 PO QID or 500 mg PO BID (for hypomagnesemia)

Magnesium oxide 140 mg PO QID or 400–500 mg PO BID (for hypomagnesemia)

Megestrol acetate (Megace) 20 mg PO BID (dose for hot flashes)

Mitomycin C 40 mg in 40 cc sterile water or NS intravesical q week for 8 weeks (therapeutic dose)

Nilutamide (Nilandron) 300 mg PO q day for 30 days, then 150 mg PO q day thereafter (for combined androgen deprivation for prostate cancer)

Oxybutynin (Ditropan XL) 5 mg PO q day to 25 mg PO q day (for urge incontinence)

Potassium citrate 20 mEq PO TID (for stone disease)

Phenazopyridine (Pyridium) 200 mg PO TID (for urinary tract infection)

Sildenafil (Viagra) 50–100 mg 1 hour prior to sexual intercourse (for erectile dysfunction)

Tadalafil (Cialis) 10–20 mg 1 hour prior to sexual intercourse (for erectile dysfunction)

Tamsulosin (Flomax) 0.4 mg PO qHS (for benign prostate hyperplasia)

Terazosin (Hytrin) 1 mg to 10 mg PO qHS (for benign prostate hyperplasia)

Testosterone enanthate or testosterone cypionate 200–300 mg IM q 2 to 3 weeks (adjust based on testosterone levels) (for benign prostate hyperplasia)

Thiola TM 1–2 g per day divided QID (for cystinuria)

Thiotepa 30 mg in 30 cc of normal saline instilled intravesically each week for 6 to 8 weeks (usual therapeutic dose) (for bladder cancer)

Tolterodine (Detrol LA) 2 mg and 4 mg, PO q day (for overactive bladder)

Vardenafil (Levitra) 5–20 mg 1 hour prior to sexual intercourse (for erectile dysfunction)

Vitamin E 1000–1500 IU PO q day (for Peyronie's disease)

Yohimbine 5.4 mg PO TID (for erectile dysfunction)

PEDIATRIC DOSES OF COMMONLY USED MEDICATIONS

Nitrofurantoin PO 5–7 mg/kg per day divided QID (for UTI); 1.5 mg/kg per day (for suppressive therapy)

Oxybutynin (Ditropan) elixir 5 mg per 5 cc PO, 0.1 mg/kg per dose BID or TID

Phenazopyridine (Pyridium) PO 12 mg/kg per day divided TID (used in patients >6 years old)

Thiola PO 15 mg/kg per day divided QID (for cystinuria)

Trimethoprim-sulfamethoxazole elixir: therapeutic dose = 8 mg trimethoprim and 40 mg sulfamethoxazole per kg per day, divided BID

Index

Note: Page numbers followed by f refer to figures; those followed by t refer to tables; those followed by b refer to boxes.